The Brainy Athlete

Published by Grammar Factory Publishing, an imprint of MacMillan Company Limited.
Permission is granted to electronically copy and to print in hard copy the WOW grading sheets provided in this book for the sole purpose of use in the WOW system. Any other use of WOW grading sheets or other materials in this book, except in the case of brief passages quoted in a book review or article, without the prior written permission of the author is strictly prohibited, including reproduction for purposes other than those noted above, sale for any purpose, modification, distribution, or republication. All enquiries should be made to the author.

Grammar Factory Publishing
MacMillan Company Limited
25 Telegram Mews, 39th Floor, Suite 3906
Toronto, Ontario, Canada
M5V 3Z1

www.grammarfactory.com

Mills, Gaz.
The Brainy Athlete: Prioritise Your Brain to Improve Your Performance and Wellbeing / Gaz Mills.

Paperback ISBN 978-1-998756-25-4
Hardcover ISBN 978-1-998756-30-8
eBook ISBN 978-1-998756-26-1
Audiobook ISBN 978-1-998756-29-2

1. SPO047000 SPORTS & RECREATION / Training. 2. SPO041000 SPORTS & RECREATION / Sports Psychology. 3. HEA000000 HEALTH & FITNESS / General.

Production Credits
Cover design by Designerbility
Interior layout design by Dania Zafar
Book production and editorial services by Grammar Factory Publishing
internal illustrations by Sophia Meldrum Designs

Grammar Factory's Carbon Neutral Publishing Commitment
Grammar Factory Publishing is proud to be neutralising the carbon footprint of all printed copies of its authors' books printed by or ordered directly through Grammar Factory or its affiliated companies through the purchase of Gold Standard-Certified International Offsets.

Disclaimer
The material in this publication is of the nature of general comment only and does not represent professional advice. It is not intended to provide specific guidance for particular circumstances, and it should not be relied on as the basis for any decision to take action or not take action on any matter which it covers. Readers should obtain professional advice where appropriate, before making any such decision. To the maximum extent permitted by law, the author and publisher disclaim all responsibility and liability to any person, arising directly or indirectly from any person taking or not taking action based on the information in this publication.

The Brainy Athlete

Prioritise your brain to improve your performance and wellbeing!

Gaz Mills

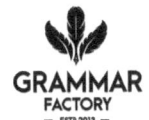

GRAMMAR FACTORY
— EST⁰ 2013 —

Testimonials

'Gaz's insights and techniques have brought me in tune with my brain and where it needs to be to allow my best self to shine through on the field. Gaz's approach has undoubtedly helped shape the player I am today. This book will help you experience the best of yourself and your performances.'

Maitlan Brown

Professional Cricketer, NSW Breakers & Sydney Sixers, Australia

'*The Brainy Athlete* is like no book I have read before and delves into an area I know so many athletes lack awareness and true understanding of. Gaz communicates complex, evidence-based neuroscience in easy language and will get you re-thinking your relationship with your brain in a powerful way. This is a book I will regularly utilise myself and recommend to all my athletes!'

Dave Halpin

Accredited Exercise Physiologist & Exercise Scientist, Ultraman & 7 x Ironman finisher, triathlon & running coach

'Success in my age group at the Ironman World Championships has not come easily and I have had many setbacks. I have sought coaching and guidance for my physical condition but I hadn't thought of my mental state or brain energy. This book really resonates with me and gave me a giggle, and your first brainy decision is to get this book to uncover the secrets to more purposeful and fulfilling sporting success.'

Angela Ballerini

3 x Ironman World Championship triathlete, multiple age-group triathlon winner, busy corporate professional

'An athlete's brain is the most important tool they have. Gaz helps athletes understand their relationship with their brain and its power in giving them the best chance of success both on and off the racecourse.'

James Thorp
Former professional triathlete and head performance triathlon coach

'*The Brainy Athlete* is easy reading and thought-provoking. Gaz Mills inspires gentle shifts in our day-to-day training and living habits by generously sharing his own vulnerabilities, experiences and research towards a stronger and holistic approach to being your best self.'

Vikki Fischer
Mother, former elite athlete, senior executive and ACT Brumbies board member

'I cannot afford to ignore the brain's role in the mind-body connection, so having an easy to read, neuroscience-based book that focuses on becoming a "Brainy Athlete" is a fantastic resource. Gaz provides an excellent set of practical and effective brain-loving strategies that support peak athletic performance as well as the enjoyment of a dynamic, fulfilling life.'

Dr Martin Fryer
Nerve/muscle scientist, ultramarathon running legend and coach, Australian Ultrarunning Hall of Fame, 2023

'Gaz's *Brainy Athlete* approach has been awesome at helping me look after my brain and mindset to give the best account of myself. It helped me to find "me" on the cricket field again.'

Tammy Beaumont, MBE

Professional Cricketer, Kent and England, 2021 ICC Women's T20 Cricketer of the Year

'As a past Olympian, I understand the importance of being in the right mindset to maximise performance, but this is an area where I could have worked more to be a better athlete. Gaz, through research and storytelling, has constructed this book as a tool for you, the athlete, to maximise your performance with winning strategies that will help you get the edge on your competition.'

Megan Hall

Olympic athlete 2004, Paralympic triathlon coach Tokyo, 2020 Mum to two beautiful children and wife to Mal

Dedication

The Brainy Athlete is dedicated to our miniature schnauzer, Sachi, who we lost while this book was going through the publishing process.

Our little girl was my wife's best mate, my office buddy, and deeply loved by all our family.

Sachi showed us life's simple pleasures are often all our brain needs to feel alive, happy and well.

Sachi, you are forever in our memories and hearts. xxx

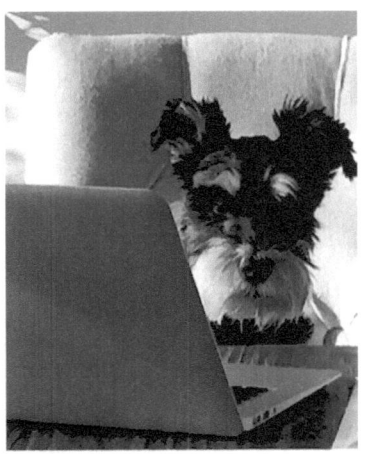

Sachi

2007 – 2023

Contents

A Note to You, the Reader

Being an athlete and watching sport are big parts of my life. I grew up with cricket and football and followed this up as a rower, endurance triathlete, and now, predominantly, I'm a cyclist. Yes, I'm comfortable admitting there is a Lycra® trend there in my last three sports, but it's more of a coincidence than purposely planned. I do love the feel of spandex, though.

I began coaching elite and professional athletes on their mental game a few years ago. Since then, I have developed a deeper understanding of them and their world. I was never an elite-level athlete or a pro, but what I love more than playing or watching sports is helping athletes at all levels achieve their best brain performance so they can perform closer to their best at training and in competition. I fell in love with my brain a few years ago, and I want you to experience the same connection to yours.

....

It's the only brain you'll ever have; how you treat it can make or break you as an athlete.

....

Australian cricketer Maitlan Brown was the first professional athlete who trusted me to help her become more in tune with her brain to improve her performance and mental game. She currently plays for the Sydney Sixers and New South Wales Breakers and has represented her country. Maitlan loves cricket and life, which shows in everything she does. She is world-class on and off the field and is a fine example of how we can never stop learning and growing as athletes and people.

After working with Maitlan for a few weeks, she described her progress like this, 'So far it's been awesome. I'm noticing a clearer mindset around training and a deeper understanding of my development as both a player and a person.' I continue to support Maitlan when she needs it, but it's much less these days because she has learned a lot about herself and prioritising her brain's care, and she performs very well in her mental game. As a result, her performances are more consistent, exciting and rewarding. I'm relieved I'm not facing her deliveries or bowling to her.

Working with elite and professional athletes broke new ground for me. Prior to that I had been coaching and developing leaders and teams in the corporate and government sectors. Yet in other ways it wasn't anything new to me, because world-class athletes are humans too and have brains just the same as leaders in any workplace. Also, where professional athletes train and compete is their workplace, just like an executive office building is a corporate leader's workplace.

As an athlete you train your body, practise your technical skills, work on your mental strength, and learn the rules and tactics of your sport. It's drummed into you that you must allow time for your body to rest and recover to become fitter, faster and stronger. If you don't, your body will be at risk of being overtrained, you may feel extra fatigued, your performance will probably suffer, and you may even stop enjoying your sport.

....

Our brain commonly suffers from the 'out of sight, out of mind' principle.

....

Our brains are hidden inside our skull our whole life, so unlike our physical appearance and performance, we can't observe our brain's form by looking in the mirror, jumping on the scales, or comparing today's run time recorded on our sport watch to our personal best. It's too easy for us to pay more attention to our bodies at the expense of our brain, which is unhelpful because we rely on their shared connection to survive and thrive.

Our busy lifestyles and many daily choices also impact our brain's performance because we're working our brain harder than we need to or should be. We use precious energy reserves we may need later, and our brain doesn't effectively recover because we don't fully appreciate how it affects everything we do as athletes, its biological limitations, and what it needs. Neglecting your brain jeopardises everything you work hard at almost every day to become a better athlete.

In this book, you will find practical steps to help you take better care of your brain so it can do its most important job: look after your body. They can help you during and between your training or competitions and have helped athletes and non-athlete humans alike.

....

Treasure your brain by building a stronger and more loving relationship with it.

....

But this book isn't just a collection of strategies to help your brain rest and recover. I want to challenge you to change how you think about your brain. Because I intentionally shifted my relationship with my brain from mostly being 'out of sight, out of mind' to becoming front of mind, I feel more energised, motivated and alive. I am a better athlete and human because I love my brain, and I feel like my brain loves me back more than it ever has.

It's important that you know that while I am a qualified professional coach and have studied neuroscience, I'm not medically qualified to provide advice on any mental or physical health issues, which is not my intention for this book. Instead, my intent has been to simplify brain science and add some stories, case studies, research, opinions and humour to understand your brain, along with some practical strategies to help you actively take care of it. When you do this, you will become a Brainy Athlete who prioritises your brain to improve your performance and wellbeing.

When you decide to become a Brainy Athlete, you will have a clearer mind and more energy to perform closer to your best. Your brain will have more cognitive resources available to deal with the challenges you face that can overwhelm an exhausted brain.

Brainy Athletes understand that to get the best from their brain, they need to give their best when looking after it. It's time to take your brain on a journey. I hope you will fall in love with yours and become a Brainy Athlete.

The Hectic Athlete

The cost to your performance

When your life is hectic, your biggest challenge is that so much is competing for your time, energy and attention – 24/7. It feels like a full calendar with work, relationships, family, jobs at home, and travelling from A to Z. Balancing your busy life can be exhausting.

Life can feel at times like your mind is swirling around in a washing machine. If you're a triathlete, it can feel like a mass swim start where, in the space of two minutes, you get hit in the face, panic, get angry, kick someone in the head accidentally (or maybe not), all while thinking you're going to die or questioning why you keep doing this to yourself.

But you survive and keep returning for more when that race is finally over, just like life.

....

As if you didn't have a lot on your plate already! But at some stage you decided, were encouraged or were fooled into becoming an amateur or elite working athlete.

....

This means that you not only train and compete for hours every week in your sport, but you must also fit this around everything else you do.

Your athletic passion is much more than a hobby to you or something you only do now and then. You do more than go to the gym or for a walk a couple of times a week – not that I'm being critical of those routines because it's still doing something active; however, your athletic commitments involve a lot more training, effort and time. Depending on your sport, you may have spent a small fortune on gear, travel, nutrition, insurance, memberships, coaching and race registrations.

When you're not actually training or competing, you spend a lot of your waking hours thinking about your sport, watching YouTube clips from experts or pro athletes, and drooling over new gear or gadgets online. You've probably got a coach, had one before, are thinking about getting one for the first time, or maybe you bought a program online.

....

Unless people you know are also into fitness and sport, they probably find you boring or crazy, or don't understand you.

....

Maybe you enjoy being part of an athlete squad, team or community. Perhaps the solo experience is your preference, where it's just you, your environment, your own thoughts, and nobody annoying you with small talk. Like me, you might enjoy a mix of group and alone time because sometimes you like people, and at other times you don't, or they don't like you.

You probably get a little too excited when someone mentions Zwift, TrainingPeaks, Strava, Garmin, Whoop, or any other gear and gadgets related to your sport. Unless people you know also share this passion, they probably find you boring or crazy, or don't know what you're talking about half the time. That's a big reason why you love your community of like-minded athletes. They get you, and you get them.

You train most days of the week, sometimes more than once a day, and compete at amateur, age-group or elite events. You love your sport and probably want to do it more, but life gets in the way, or it doesn't pay you enough. The hectic pace often feels mentally and physically fatiguing.

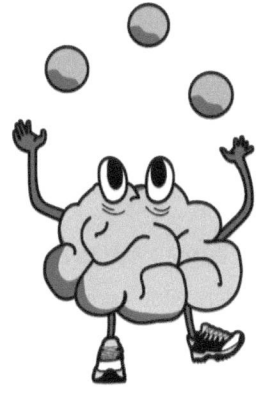

You're juggling your professional and personal life to pursue your fitness and sports goals, but it often feels like you're juggling more balls than you can handle.

As an athlete, you've learned that if you don't allow your body to rest, recover and recharge, you can feel physically exhausted, and your performance and enjoyment of your sport will suffer. Your fitness and performance stall, drop, or even free fall when you don't care for your body by managing its energy and fatigue.

There's a tonne of information out there to help you rest and recharge your body, and like me, you probably have a couple (or a dozen) books on this topic. My cycling coach says, 'You get faster when you're resting and recovering, not when you're working hard.' Of course, I must work hard to improve as an athlete, but without including down time and easy efforts in my training to allow my body to recover and recharge, I feel exhausted, and my performance suffers.

....

I take a different approach to help you rest, recover and recharge by focusing on your brain's needs to help you become a Brainy Athlete.

....

But it's not only your body you need to take care of to be your fittest and healthiest as an athlete and, more importantly, a human.

YOUR BRAIN RUNS EVERYTHING

Your body may perform the physical movements that allow you to do some awesome action moves on the field, track, course, water, soft floor, mountains or stadium, but your brain is in charge and needs to be fit and well too.

Just like your muscles need energy to run, climb, cycle, lift, jump, bounce, ski, row, kick, throw, flip, hop and swim, your brain needs energy to collect, process and interpret millions of bits of information every second, most of which happens without you being aware of it.

....

*Your brain uses more energy than
any other part of your body.*

....

Your brain requires a lot of energy because it uses more than any other body part, including your spring-loaded quads, massive biceps or ripped six-pack. On average, an adult brain only weighs two to three per cent of your body weight, but consumes around twenty per cent of your total energy. Your brain includes between 80 and 100 billion neurons, or nerve cells, which communicate with each other via trillions of electrical and chemical signals travelling across your brain and central nervous system.

....

*'Your brain's most important job is to control your
body, so you stay alive and well.'*
–DR LISA FELDMAN BARRETT

....

Dr Lisa Feldman Barrett has published over 260 peer-reviewed scientific papers and is in the top one per cent of most cited scientists worldwide for her ground-breaking research in psychology and neuroscience. Dr Barrett explains that your 'brain's most important job is to control your body, so you stay alive and well' by controlling and coordinating your body's systems 'as they burn and replenish energy efficiently.' [1]

Dr Barrett says if you eat healthily, have quality sleep and exercise regularly, 'your brain won't have to work as hard' to keep your body in balance.[2] Your brain and body are co-dependent systems, and when you take care of both, you support your whole internal system. Building on Dr Barrett's expertise, it's clear to me that we must prioritise our brain to be healthy, fulfilled and able to perform at our athletic best. This is undeniable.

....

My theory is that our most important job is caring for our brain so it can effectively do its most important job: looking after our body.

....

When your body needs to rest and recover, your brain will make decisions based on those needs because that's its most important job. When you feel extra tired or sore, you speak to your coach, adjust some training, have extra rest or seek medical advice. But how often do you take this recovery approach when your brain feels low on energy? You know the uncomfortable feeling of forcing yourself to keep going when you're mentally and physically spent. It happens in our workplaces, at home, dragging ourselves up a flight of stairs because the escalator is broken, or deciding what to have for dinner at 7 pm. Like many people, your strategy is usually to push on and go to bed exhausted – day after day.

As an athlete, when your brain is fatigued or feels low on energy, it's harder and sometimes feels impossible to mentally push through and deliver the performances you know your body can achieve. When your brain is spent, it's harder to manage the stress and worry that comes with life's busy, uncertain and fast-moving pace.

FATIGUE IMPACTS YOUR BRAIN AND BODY PERFORMANCE

A 2018 study on the effect of mental fatigue on cognitive and aerobic performance for endurance athletes found that 'mental fatigue impairs whole-body endurance and cognitive performance.' The researchers said this has 'subjective, behavioural, and physiological' indicators produced 'by prolonged periods of demanding cognitive activity.' [3] This means that when your brain works harder for longer, you don't just feel fatigued; both your behaviour and biology change too.

When you exercise, you experience fatigue from your muscles (peripheral fatigue) or from your central nervous system (central fatigue), which is your brain and spinal cord. Your tired feeling can be the result of peripheral, central or both types of fatigue. Central fatigue is believed to happen when the signals between your neurons become weak and 'your muscles will not be able to contract at their strongest, even when you think you are using them to their maximum.' [5] The time of recovery from central fatigue can vary from one minute to days, depending on the modality, duration and intensity of exercise.[6] Prioritising your brain's rest and recovery is essential to experience your best physical performance.

A 2009 study on the effect mental fatigue has on physical endurance found that when these athletes 'performed a mentally fatiguing task before a difficult exercise test, they reached exhaustion more quickly than when they did the same exercise when mentally rested.' Importantly, researchers observed that the athletes' 'mental fatigue did not cause the heart or muscles to perform differently.' [6] The point at which they reached exhaustion was determined by their perceived effort, which means their brain felt like the physical effort was harder even though their body was not working harder than usual. The same study also found the athletes' concentration and attention to their performance were impaired when their brain was fatigued.

....

Athletes reached exhaustion more quickly than when they did the same exercise when mentally rested.

....

Learning and retaining new skills and techniques to improve your athletic brain and abilities is harder. Dr Barrett says, 'When you're exposed to new and different things, your brain works a bit harder than usual. Your neurons require more resources when you're learning, such as water, salt, glucose, and various other chemicals.'[7] Your brain is using more fuel when it works harder, just like your car does when you put the foot down on the accelerator to drive up a steep hill. The extra energy being burned by your brain isn't substantial, but it's enough to have an impact over time, particularly if you don't replenish your energy.

'One important thing to remember is the most expensive things that your brain can do are move your body, like exercise, right? And learning something new,' says Dr Barrett. 'There always comes a point where it's kind of unpleasant. You're tired and struggling, and you have to push through that. It's true with exercise; it's true with learning.'[8]

....

If your brain is low on energy before you start your training session or a race, it's harder to push through to perform so that you get the best return on your time and effort.

....

Brain fatigue will happen when you push yourself physically because you burn energy, but if you're already fatigued before you start, you will hit the wall quicker and ease up earlier. You know from your own performances that a mentally fatigued athlete is typically slower to react, misses important cues and information, sucks at planning on the run, can't adapt well to unexpected changes, is less tolerant of other people, struggles more with pressure and stress, and can be less committed to enduring the discomfort that goes with physically pushing yourself.

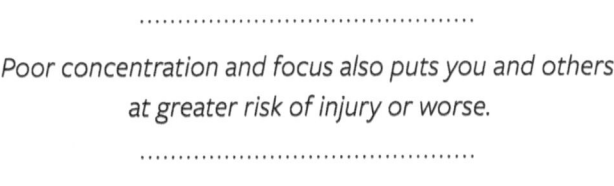

Poor concentration and focus also puts you and others at greater risk of injury or worse.

Being mentally rested and switched on is not just an objective for improving your performance. Poor concentration and decisions also put you and others at greater risk of injury or worse. This is very dangerous if you do sports like cycling, rock climbing, trail running, CrossFit, auto racing, sky diving, gymnastics, shooting or parkour.

Another reason that can help explain why your brain lets you know when it's fatigued comes from Claude Messier, a Canadian Professor, who studies how the brain uses lactate and glucose to fuel its activities.

During an interview with the publication *Scientific American*, Messier explains, 'The brain has a hard time staying focused on just one thing for too long.'[9] Messier has a theory wherein he says, 'It's possible that sustained concentration creates some changes in the brain that promote avoidance of that state. It could be like a timer that says, "Okay you're done now.'"

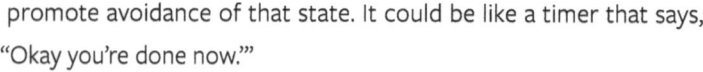

'Maybe the brain just doesn't like to work so hard for so long.'
– PROFESSOR CLAUDE MESSIER

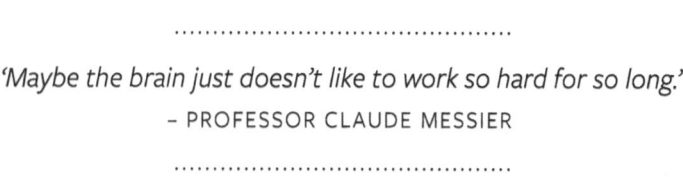

While it's not proven, Messier's theory is one reasonable explanation for why you may find it hard to continue concentrating without having breaks to do something that's less taxing to freshen up your brain. It may help explain why you may lose concentration or effort after doing something for a while. This may also help explain why we can stay tuned into something we're interested in for hours, while we can zone out after five seconds when we're not.

I found this theory relatable to both the full Ironman races I've done. At around the 120km mark of the 180km bike leg, my brain went through a stage of having enough and wanting to do something else. I wasn't physically exhausted, but my brain was over being on the bike, even though I love cycling. This is a very different experience from when I'm physically at my limit, and I just want the race or training session to be over.

Whether fatigue is caused by your brain using more energy to work harder, losing interest, or not recovering from whatever happened earlier, you will know when your brain feels fatigued. (Fig 1) The why isn't necessarily the most important question to ask because you may never know why you're feeling tired, or it could be a combination of things.

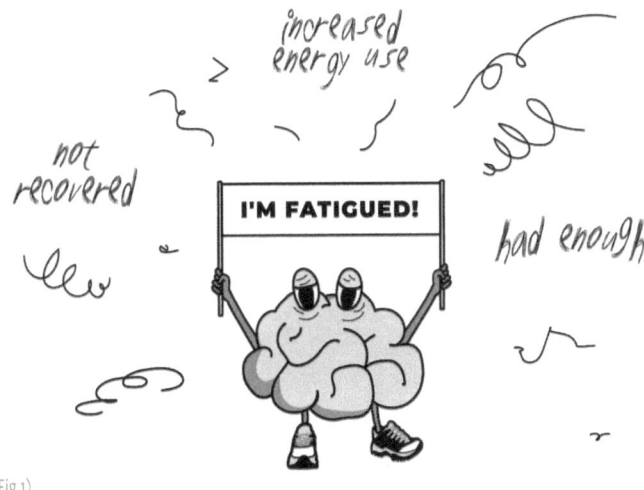

(Fig 1)

A more helpful question to ask can be, 'What?' What can you do to help your brain rest and recover? This book will help you answer that question. When you make better choices for your brain, you should start feeling mental, emotional and physical benefits. However, if it's an ongoing issue or it doesn't improve, I encourage you to seek medical help because it may be more than just your brain feeling fatigued.

OUT OF SIGHT, OUT OF MIND

I believe one big barrier to effectively managing your brain is the 'out of sight, out of mind' principle. Your brain is always hidden inside your protective skull, which is a good thing for your ongoing survival, but a downside is that we don't pay enough attention to it.

....

Your hidden brain is often not on your mind, which is ironic considering your brain creates your mind.

....

When things are not on your mind, they are not a priority, and for your brain, this means you can neglect its needs. As a result, you may suffer tiring consequences. The fact that you're reading this means you're keen to make your brain's fitness and health a stronger priority, which is awesome for you, your brain, and your passion for your sport.

Just like you have helpful strategies for improving your physical performance, you need to make sure your brain is on your mind if you're going to improve your physical and mental performance. This book deliberately targets what your brain needs because it's usually forgotten, neglected, or not understood or prioritised compared to how much attention is paid to your physical goals, development and achievements. Your brain and body are complex and co-dependent systems, so whatever strategies you apply will have some effect on both.

....

Changes in our brain are less obvious and much harder to measure than our physical goals, development and achievements.

....

We're quick to notice changes in our body shape, muscles, weight, data, and other observations or information that influence our athletic performances. We notice it in the mirror, at weigh-in time, on our watches, bike computers and video footage, in the weight we lift, and by analysing streams of data downloaded on our computers.

There's no shortage of gadgets, gear and information to help you physically perform and recover. You can instantly measure your heart rate, pace or power to make decisions during training and racing. We measure these details over time to help us plan and analyse our training, often with a coach, which includes rest and recovery to avoid overtraining, injuries, excessive fatigue and a drop in performance.

....

*We're spoiled for choice in the
physical recovery market.*

....

For example, we can buy leg compression gadgets for fresher legs and electric massage guns to smooth out our sore muscles – and unintentionally scare our pets because it sounds like a jackhammer on a construction site! I use the massage gun and a freezing ice bath or dip in the cold ocean to help my body recover. The cold water also trains my brain to be calmer and control my breathing, which helps when I'm feeling anxious or highly stressed as an athlete.

So, what does the consumer market look like for our brain? Technology that's helped me take care of my brain's fitness and improve its performance is readily available. However, the market has a limited and narrow range when you compare it to the thousands of products readily available to support your body's performance. In other chapters, I talk about a couple of funky gadgets I've used that have helped with my brain's fitness, wellbeing and performance.

THERE IS NO OFF SWITCH

You may have read or heard that humans only use ten per cent of their brains. That is a myth, even though sometimes you may feel like you're only using five per cent, or you're sure someone you're talking to is using just one per cent. It's realistic to assume that none of us will ever realise 100 per cent of our brain's potential for various reasons, but that doesn't mean we need to be at 100 per cent performance to succeed as athletes or in any other area of life. Perfection is not your goal; being your best is.

We can't say with certainty how close any of us are to using our brain's full potential because it's such a complex question and there are so many unknown variables. However, we struggle more, mentally and physically, when our brain is exhausted than when our brain feels rested and energised.

Your whole brain does something every second of the day until it dies. Even in deep restorative sleep, your brain does internal housework to repair and restore itself, while REM sleep includes dreaming and sorting what's worth keeping from the day and what can be tossed in the bin. When I don't get enough of this good sleep, I can feel mentally foggy. It's harder to concentrate, I can forget what happened yesterday, and I can also be a bit grumpy.

....

Your brain is never not thinking or turned off, so you're mentally active a lot more than you're physically active.

....

Your brain is never not thinking or turned off. Even in a deep sleep, your brain is working and processing thoughts. This means you're mentally active a lot more than you're physically active. You might train your body a couple of hours a day, and even if you overdo a session, there are still twenty-two hours in the day where you're not pushing your body other than counting your steps on your fitness watch.

The Neuroleadership Institute is a global brain research company that specialises in organisational performance. They explain that 'As living organisms, our brains are subject to natural biological limits that significantly benefit from frequent, mindful breaks to maximise attentional resources and manage stress.'[10]

If you want to put yourself in a stronger position to experience the best of your skills, grit, focus, planning, enjoyment, agility and performance as an athlete, without doubt, you must prioritise your brain's care. This book will help you manage the flow of energy and fatigue you experience so you can perform closer to your athletic best. You will experience brain fatigue and have off days, but your brainier choices and actions will have more influence over how fit your brain is feeling.

....

The answers you're looking for to become a Brainy Athlete are not rocket science. They're brain science, and you'll find many of them in this book.

....

To be the best athlete you can be, your brain needs the energy to think critically under pressure, make good decisions, regulate your emotions, outsmart your worries and fears, be in tune with your body, remain calm, and come up with a new plan when your original plan is no longer working. These problems are real for all athletes and can happen suddenly and unexpectedly during training, competition and anywhere else in life. Brainy athletes can use their brains more effectively because they are more effective at caring for their brains. The answers you're looking for to become a Brainy Athlete are not rocket science. They're brain science, and you'll find many of them in this book.

INTRODUCTION HIGHLIGHTS

1. Your brain requires a lot of energy because it uses more than any other part of your body.
2. Your brain and body are complex and co-dependent systems; however, your brain can suffer from the 'out of sight, out of mind' principle.
3. If your brain feels low on energy before you train and compete, it's harder to push through and studies have shown that athletes reach exhaustion quicker.
4. Our most important job is caring for our brain so it can effectively do its most important job: looking after our body.
5. Perfection is not your goal; prioritisation is.

Chapter 1

The Brain Energy Continuum

Your brain's energy flow

I never used to be a morning person, but that's changed. I love getting up early, around 5:30 am, and if I'm not training straight away, I'll get a couple of hours of work in before getting on my bike for the day's session. You may have heard the phrase 'win the morning, win the day' or something similar. For me, this is true. I feel energised when I first get up and use that energy to kickstart the day. That is unless I've had a late night, alcohol, a restless sleep, I feel sick, or any other reason my brain feels fatigued. But most mornings I feel energised and motivated, and I am convinced that's because I take much better care of my brain the day before and regularly end the day with a good sleep routine.

....

When I'm energised in the morning, it's a great time for me to focus on challenging or complex work, and it's also a great time for me to get creative.

....

My energy continues to be up throughout the morning if I feed my brain and take mini breaks to give it some downtime to refresh. For example, I've written a lot of this book in the first hours of the day because my mind is clear and the thoughts flow, which was necessary for me to work around my business. Typically, mid-afternoon is the Achilles heel for my brain's energy. I usually don't feel sharp when I do complex or creative work in the afternoon. Instead, I'll pick easier tasks like admin, or I'll have a complete break from work and do something else. Then, I usually get a second wind later in the afternoon, and if I've taken a couple of hours off in the afternoon, I'll often do some work in the evening.

It doesn't always work out this way, but my brain's energy flow is pretty consistent if I'm also consistent at caring for my brain. Your brain's energy flow may be different from mine or could be similar. Remember that every brain is unique, but all brains will be affected by how we manage our energy needs and rest; in my experience, we can change how our brains flow by how we take care of them. Once I started taking better care of my brain with a better sleep routine, mini breaks and better nutrition, I stopped having my regular afternoon naps. The mid-afternoon is still my least creative period; however, I am still productive and don't need a nap. I am more in tune with my brain's energy flow because I have prioritised its needs, and while I do still experience fatigue like we all do, it's not as deep and doesn't last as long.

....

*We all have times when our brains don't want to play,
and we may not know why.*

....

Think about a time when your body was feeling good enough for what you needed to do, but mentally you were tired, foggy, confused, indecisive, or just couldn't be bothered. Maybe your brain was resisting because it needed to recover from something that happened before-hand. This could have been a poor sleep, a long day at work, too much time looking at your phone, or maybe you didn't eat or drink well enough the day before. What you do for your brain in recent hours and even days can affect your brain's performance in the present.

If you're training smart and following a good program that includes rest days and easier sessions, your body will have loads of time to rest and recover before the next session. If you have a coach, they generally get annoyed if you overtrain by going too hard or sneaking in some extra sessions. Even if you hide your sneaky sessions from your coach by not uploading them, you can't hide from the effects this has on your recovery.

Now compare that to your current training program for your brain. If you're like most people, it's going to be unwritten, loose, largely unplanned, overlooked, and lacking enough helpful breaks.

....

We simply don't give our brain the same priority and love as we do to training and resting our body because it's out of sight and out of mind.

....

Think about how often you let your brain recover and recharge so it can perform for you in all areas of your life, not just as an athlete. We understand enough from science, research, case studies and people's experiences that there are positive actions we can all take to help our brain rest and recover for our performance and health.

Just like our race or game strategy, when we get our brain strategy and execution right, it's an amazing feeling, and we can achieve great things; however, when we get it wrong, our brain suffers, and so do we. Generally, we feel somewhere in between.

INFLUENCING YOUR BRAIN'S ENERGY FLOW

I created the Brain Energy Continuum (BEC) (Fig 2) as a simple way to show that our brain's energy flow fluctuates and, as a result, our cognitive and physical performance will too. It's a simple visual that helps to explain the impact of our choices, things beyond our control, and influences we don't fully understand or know about our brain and body. Where your brain's energy is located on the BEC right now will influence its ability to process this chapter and understand what I'm explaining to you.

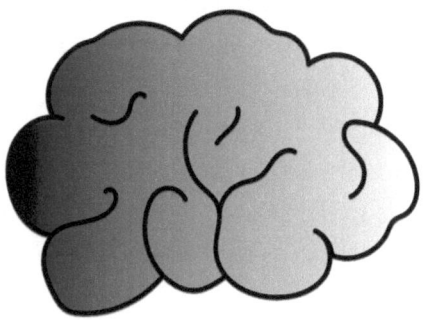

EXHAUSTED   ENERGISED

- *Lacking energy*   - *Strong energy*
- *Drowsy*   - *Focused*
- *Moody*   - *Calm*
- *Inattentive*   - *Alert*
- *Unmotivated*   - *Active*

(Fig 2) Brain Energy Continuum

My idea to create the BEC came from the mental health continuum I became familiar with as a speaker for the Australian mental health organisation, Beyond Blue. The mental health continuum is described as 'a range or a continuum where mental health is at one end, represented by feeling good and functioning well, through to severe symptoms of mental health conditions at the other. Mental health is not fixed or in a static state, and we can move back and forth along this scale at different times during our lives.' [14]

Applying a similar concept to your brain's energy flow makes sense to me because at one end of the BEC, you feel like you can take on the world or break your previous personal best. On the opposite end, you feel completely exhausted and motionless.

....

Most of the time, you find yourself somewhere between the two ends of the BEC.

....

If you fuel your brain well during the day and get a solid night's sleep, your brain will likely feel well rested and energised for an early morning training session the next day. If you're feeling like this, you may be closer to the 'energised' or right side of the BEC. Alternatively, if you stay up late, have a few wines or beers, and have a restless sleep, you'll likely find yourself closer to the 'exhausted' or left side. You may still get your session done, but how effective will you be, and how will you feel afterwards?

....

It's not too late to start making better choices for your brain's energy flow.

....

The changes to my sleep and nutrition at the start of this chapter are two reasons why I am consistently living closer to the energised end of the BEC. The BEC is a tool to remind you that your choices create consequences that impact your brain and performance. You can decide if you're happy to accept those consequences. If you're not, you can choose differently, and once you put those choices into action, you can experience different results.

If you decide you want to live your life closer to the 'energised' side of the BEC and put what you learn from this book into action, you'll have chosen to become a Brainy Athlete, and your brain will love you for that.

A colour version of the BEC and your access to other Brainy Athlete resources is on my website at gazmills.com/brainyresources.

BRAIN FATIGUE & IMPULSE

Glutamate is an abundant neurotransmitter in your brain and sends chemical messages between your brain's neurons to help them communicate with each other. Glutamate is critical to your learning and memory, and can be used as an energy source by your brain. The Cleveland Clinic health and medical research centre explains, 'For your brain to function properly, glutamate needs to be present in the right concentration in the right places at the right time.' Too little is thought to lead to impaired concentration, brain exhaustion and low energy.[11] Excessive levels of glutamate in the brain can cause brain cell damage and are associated with some serious health conditions.

A 2022 study identified a link between brain function and a chemical change in participants' brains while they put their brains to work in front of computers. Forty participants were split into two groups for the study, and each person performed tasks on a computer screen that involved memory and economic decisions. [12] [13]

One group performed mentally challenging tasks, while the other group had similar but mentally easier tasks. Both groups worked for six hours and had only two ten-minute breaks during that time. It doesn't sound like a nice place to work.

Neuroscientists monitored the groups' brains while they worked, focusing on the level of glutamate in an area of the brain important to decision-making and impulse control. They identified that the harder working group had higher levels of glutamate for longer than the group taking things easy. These results indicate that:

- when the brain must reduce the high levels of glutamate hanging around after working harder, it reduces participants' control over their impulsive decision-making, and they choose low-effort options
- it can feel harder to use our thinking caps effectively at the end of a 'strenuous' workday

This all means that when you work your brain harder before you train or compete, changes in your brain's chemistry may lead you to make impulsive and lazy decisions that can hurt your strategy and athletic performance.

CHAPTER HIGHLIGHTS

1. Your brain's energy flow and fatigue levels fluctuate, and you won't always understand why.
2. The choices you make every day play a critical role in how energised you feel and how well you perform.
3. You may still get your session done with a fatigued brain, but how effective will you be, and how will you feel afterwards?
4. The BEC is a tool to remind you that your choices create consequences that impact your brain and performance.
5. It's not too late to start making better choices for your brain's energy flow.

Chapter 2

Become a Brainy Athlete

Prioritise your brain to feel more energised, motivated and alive!

In my mid-thirties, I worked in a specialist policing role where we had to maintain a high level of physical fitness to remain operational. Almost every workday, we had physical training scheduled in the gym and outdoors. It was hard and painful at times, but being part of a team in this environment was great. This experience was a lot like being in a high-performance sports team where, together, you train at work, experience the ups and downs, share success and disappointment, make mistakes, learn a lot, and form a team bond that is hard to replicate outside of these environments.

Like my rowing, triathlon and cycling experiences over the years, how well I played the mental or brain game in this policing role was just as important as how physically fit and strong I was. In fact, there were many times when my brain game was most important because making good decisions and maintaining focus mattered more than how far I could run or how heavy I could lift. When everyone was physically hurting, and a task still required a high level of concentration and technical skills, how well my brain was functioning played a role in determining success or failure.

....

*I knew I had to rest my body, but I don't recall explicitly
talking about prioritising my brain's rest or recovery.*

....

Physical fitness and technical skills aside, our mental strength was
regularly tested and assessed. If our mental strength wasn't up to
scratch, it showed in our performance and behaviours because there
were always people watching, and for a good reason. If we couldn't
continue to do our jobs well when things became tough, we risked
people getting hurt or failing to achieve our goals.

Mental strength means having mental strategies to continue performing
effectively when faced with hardship, challenges, adversity and setbacks.
These are critical life skills, so while I encourage you to work on these
to help you in sports and life, this book lays out many of the fundamentals that create a strong base for your mental strength and skills.

In many individual and team sports, it's not necessarily the physically
strongest, fittest or most skillful that win. The best brains in the game
on any given day are used to strike an advantage and mentally outsmart the opposition. It's best if you have a team of energised brains
working well together to be a high-performing team. Even one fatigued
brain out of sync with everyone else's brains can mean the difference
between winning and losing.

....

A team of Brainy Athletes is formidable.

....

PRIORITISATION, NOT PERFECTION, TO BE A BRAINY ATHLETE

I define a Brainy Athlete as an 'athlete who prioritises their brain and actively cares for it to improve their performance and wellbeing.' Becoming a Brainy Athlete is not about increasing your IQ or getting straight 'A's on your exams. You should indeed feel like you have more brain power and energy because you prioritise the rest, recovery and recharging of your brain, but I can't guarantee you will suddenly discover the meaning of life or understand quantum physics.

....

This book unpacks my theory that your most important job is caring for your brain so it can effectively do its most important job: looking after your body.

....

A 2018 study of amateur cyclists tested the effect of brain fatigue on their performance. The testing included a 20 km time trial (TT) that measured time, power output and the cyclists' brain activity. [15] They tested twice in a non-fatigued state to get an accurate benchmark for all cyclists. Both test results were almost identical. The cyclists did the same 20 km TT after completing a thirty-minute cognitively demanding task on a computer.

Overall results showed that the 'task-induced mental fatigue' had changed the electrical activity in the cyclists' brains during the TT. Researchers identified a decrease in the cyclists' drive and the TT performance was 'significantly impaired.' On average, they were 2.7 per cent slower, and power output was 6.5 per cent lower. Interestingly, the cyclists increased their power significantly in all testing in the last two kilometres of the TT. I'm not surprised because we always seem to find some extra energy and motivation when the finish line is close. Those finish line feels are the real deal.

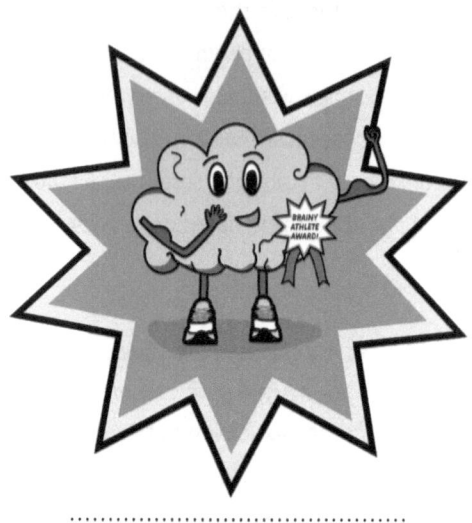

....

A Brainy Athlete is an 'athlete who prioritises their brain and actively cares for it to improve their performance and wellbeing.'

....

Becoming a Brainy Athlete begins with consciously deciding to prioritise your brain. Your brain is often out of sight, so often out of mind, which means you must keep reminding yourself it's there. Otherwise, it's easy to forget and neglect it. My computer desktop image is a brain. Not a real brain, but a computer-generated image that's pulsing with electricity and energy. That's one reminder for me. I like to gift stress balls shaped like brains to clients and program participants – that's one easy reminder for them to look after their brains.

I am a Brainy Athlete, but certainly not a perfect specimen. I have my faults and don't always get it right. Some days I don't prioritise my brain, and there are consequences – like feeling drowsy the next day, lacking energy and even being a little grumpy at times. Sometimes this is a trade-off I accept because I was at a dinner party the night before, had a few drinks, or was up late working. That's life – my brain isn't always going to feel loved, and I'm not always going to feel its love coming back. I also know that there have been many times I could have made simple choices to prioritise my brain better. My goal is to be more consistent and deliberate at caring for my brain, rather than pursuing perfection and beating myself up when I make a poor choice or stray from prioritising my brain. I learn from my experiences, accept imperfection and remain flexible because I'm not a robot.

This book has been written to help you develop a stronger connection and love for your brain. If loving your brain sounds weird, think about it this way: your brain is a partner for life, never leaves you, and is the only one you will ever have. Your brain is central to your performance, health, wellbeing, survival and success as an athlete and human.

....

You'll find practical strategies in this book that have helped my client's brains and their performances, and those clients include amateur, elite and professional athletes.

....

This book will help you lead a life with a more rested and energised brain – one that can give you more when you're:

- sweating it out in your active wear
- feeling like you're inside the pressure cooker
- solving problems
- making decisions
- dealing with injuries
- experiencing disappointments and setbacks
- going for a new PB
- feeling frightened at the start line
- screaming at your burning lungs or limbs to shut up
- needing to go deeper, harder, faster or longer
- wanting to crush your session or the competition

APPLYING THE BRAINY ATHLETE STRATEGIES

Now that you've decided to prioritise your brain, what's next? Inside this book are solutions and lifestyle strategies for your brain that help before, during and after training or competition. These strategies have helped my clients, including amateur, elite and professional athletes, improve their mental and physical performances. They also help me a lot. I consistently show my brain how much I love it; as a result, it is calmer, feels more effective, complains less about being tired, and loves me back. This has improved my quality of life in every way.

I'm confident this book can help you because neuroscience, case studies, personal experiences and research support it. Practical suggestions include prioritising your brain's care in your busy life. If they weren't practical, reading them would waste your brain's precious energy and valuable time. I deliberately haven't included a chapter on exercise and fitness because you're an athlete, so you're already doing one of the most positive and healthy behaviours for your brain and body.

You don't have to consistently practice every single strategy in this book to benefit you and your brain. Some strategies, like sleep and fuel, are necessary, while some will work better than others for your brain and be more suited to your lifestyle at different times. You don't want to make it a chore to fit everything in this book into your already busy life; some days you will be great at taking all the steps to look after your brain, and other days you won't.

I encourage you to experiment, and be persistent and consistent to discover what works best for you and your brain. Seek feedback from people after you put your strategies into action. For example, ask if they've noticed any changes in you in the last couple of weeks. Do you seem to have more energy and focus, appear less tired, be more pleasant, or be more switched on and less distracted? This external feedback can help you determine what strategies work best for you because any change in you may be more obvious to the people around you.

Quality sleep takes a big chunk out of your day, while other solutions only need moments to give your brain a rest and a burst of energy. You may already be effectively applying one or more of the strategies in this book, but there may be others that can help your brain even more.

....

You use different strategies to improve
your physical performance, now think
about your brain in the same way.

....

Some days you will need to make your brain work harder for longer, even if you don't feel like it, such as when working towards a deadline. For example, when your time and energy are under the pump at work, achievable strategies that give your brain short yet effective rest breaks during the day will set you up with a more energised brain for a training session after work.

There are also days you need to focus on your brain having a good rest, like the day before a big race or important game. A good night's sleep and fuelling your brain are probably the most important strategies for this example, which are both covered in separate chapters.

Having options up your sleeve gives you the flexibility to choose the best strategy to suit the situation and how your brain is feeling at the time. It's not easy to sleep soundly when you're freaking out the night before an early race, which is why other strategies in this book, including attention control, can help you calm your overactive brain so you can sleep and feel fresher for the big day.

....

It's best to have a selection of strategies to overcome the unpredictable events that life can throw up at any moment.

....

Your best-laid plans to have that unbroken nine-hour sleep before a big game or race can be upended by inconsiderate guests in the next hotel room, a fire alarm at 2 am, a needy child or a sick partner. Also, some days your brain doesn't want to play ball, or a strategy that usually works doesn't. If something's not working, try another strategy and see what happens. You'll never know unless you test it on yourself.

Some strategies in this book are obvious and widely promoted, but just knowing something is good for us doesn't mean we do it. When our brain is already tired, we often don't do what's good for its recovery, even if we know a particular strategy will help, because we can't be bothered with the effort involved. For example, going outside for ten minutes for a hit of fresh oxygen and some nature can feel a lot harder than sitting on our butt for three hours in front of a TV show we're half watching while scrolling through posts and stories on our phones.

Whenever we have a free moment or nothing to do, it's so easy for us to automatically reach for our phone without thinking. This has become a deep-rooted habit for many of us, but fortunately, we can rewire our brains to create better screentime habits. This is often easier said than done, but is an important strategy for improving your performance and wellbeing and is covered in *Chapter 9: Streamline Your Screentime.*

Chapter 4: Lead Your Lazy Brain explores how to influence, encourage, and sometimes drag along your lazy brain to help it recover and recharge. I've included a simple brain-friendly technique for your routines and habits, which you can use to prioritise the strategies you choose from this book.

Remember, this book isn't a magic fix for all the problems, worries, headaches, setbacks, mistakes, failures and disasters you experience as an athlete and human. These things are all part of life and can happen to the best and most experienced athletes in the world. You won't eliminate brain fatigue and if you train and play hard, you will continue to suffer mentally and physically. Nevertheless, improving your understanding of how to care for your brain will put you in a stronger position to take advantage of what your amazing brain and body can do for you and your athletic performance.

If your brain feels energised, keep reading – the next chapter is waiting for you! If your brain's feeling distracted or tired, give it a break before continuing. Simply pausing to reflect on this decision to continue or stop is a positive step you are taking to become a Brainy Athlete.

CHAPTER HIGHLIGHTS

1. A Brainy Athlete is an 'athlete who prioritises their brain and actively cares for it to improve their performance and wellbeing.' Prioritisation is not perfection.

2. This book unpacks my theory that your most important job is caring for your brain so it can effectively do its most important job: looking after your body.

3. Some days you will be great at looking after your brain, and other days you won't. Learn from this, accept imperfection and be flexible.

4. This book lays out many of the fundamentals that create a strong base for your mental strength and skills, which is having a rested and energised brain.

5. Various strategies help your physical performance; it's the same for your brain. Experiment to discover what works for you and seek feedback.

Chapter 3

Is Variety the Spice of Your Brain's Life?

Keeping your brain interested may help reduce fatigue

Chapter one opened by describing what your life as a hectic athlete may look like. You're juggling at least one sport with your work, studies, home, family, friends, and whatever else you've got going on. Or maybe your day and week look a little different to this, revolving around work or study and your sport. You may have a few activities on the go each week, or you may have only one or two that take up most of your time. Some people are consumed by their work, others don't see their work as a priority compared to their personal life, and many more are somewhere in between. Everyone is different, so everyone's brain will likely respond differently.

I've met and worked with athletes so obsessed with their sport that it takes up most of their time outside work or their studies. The reason for their obsession can vary, and they may love their sport so much that they can't switch off from it and are always looking for ways to improve. There are also athletes I've met who put huge expectations on themselves or seek perfection, so they spend most of their time working on trying to meet those expectations, which can lead to negative impacts on brain performance and health.

....

I've met and worked with athletes who are so obsessed with their sport that it takes up most of their time outside work or their studies.

....

I experienced a similar obsession with the police when my job was pretty much my entire motivation, attention and focus for several years. Everything else was secondary to my job, and even when I wasn't at work, I often thought about it in one way or another. I put my work ahead of my young family, rarely mixed outside my inner work circle, didn't have any hobbies other than exercising at the gym or running, and put too much pressure on myself. I alone created these limited boundaries. Although I might have believed I was better at my job as a result, I was generally doing more harm than good.

My brain's performance and my overall health deteriorated over time. While this book has not been written from a mental health perspective, I believe my narrow focus, lack of diversity in my lifestyle activities, and obsession with work contributed significantly to my poor mental health and depression.

....

You physically benefit from variety, and it's no different when it comes to optimising your brain's performance.

....

Lack of variety for your brain is like overtraining your body, and just because you do more of the same thing, it doesn't mean it's a good idea or that you're going to see benefits. Training your body for optimal performance is best achieved by mixing up the intensity of your workouts, varying the exercises or sets performed, including some stretching and flexibility, and resting. You physically benefit from variety, and it's no different when it comes to optimising your brain's performance.

You have probably read or heard people say you need to put everything into something to reap the rewards, seize the day, leave your legacy, become an expert, or become a superstar. While it's true that prioritisation, hard work, lifelong learning, skills development and consistency are all necessary to improve and perform to your best ability, I disagree with the notion that it's an 'all-or-nothing' approach for most people and scenarios. There are exceptions where we may need to go all out to succeed or survive, and there are people who thrive on the all-or-nothing approach. However, I don't believe this is either the norm or good for our brain. For most of us, life can be much broader and more rewarding than just putting everything into being an athlete or whatever we do for work. There is much more to life than putting all your eggs in one basket. Diversity and variety are important lifestyle choices for becoming a Brainy Athlete.

VARIETY AND DIVERSITY ARE ESSENTIAL FOR YOUR BRAIN

As a busy athlete with a hectic training schedule, you may feel like there's no room for anything else on top of what you're already doing. However, I'm now going to suggest something that could sound counter intuitive – becoming a Brainy Athlete may require adding more activities to your life, not less. This will depend on how much variety you have and if you're obsessed or occupied by only one or two things, like your work, sport or both.

If you're unsure or puzzled by my apparent madness at suggesting you can be a Brainy Athlete by including more activities unrelated to your sport in your life, consider the findings in a study published in 2021 titled, 'Change Is Good for the Brain: Activity Diversity and Cognitive Functioning Across Adulthood.'[16] This study looked at the impact diverse interests have on the brain's cognitive, executive and memory performance. To better understand the influence of various activities on the brain, researchers separated participants' interests into work, family, leisure, physical, volunteering and social categories. They also tested participants twice, with ten years between testing.

....

Cognitive, executive and memory testing on participants found that those with a variety of lifestyle activities showed higher brain performance than those with less diversity in their activities.

....

The study also showed that increasing the diversity of participants' interests over time appeared to show an improvement in their brains' performance. The findings also found that positive cognitive test results were experienced when the time spent on activities was adjusted, which means you don't necessarily need to spend a lot of time on individual activities to experience benefits. Simply switching more regularly between diverse activities can positively impact your brain's performance.

Other research quoted in this study has found that 'a variety of activities in daily life are posited [suggested] to increase cognitive reserve capacity and resilience, leading to better performance on cognitively challenging tasks.' [17][18] This means researchers have found that people with diverse activities appear to have more brain power in reserve for tackling mental challenges, which is beneficial to athletes under pressure who must make critical decisions, execute their game plan successfully, and perform.

The study also references another study that showed 'a lack of activities, or more passive behaviours such as binge TV watching, are associated with cognitive decline in older adults.' [19] While I'm not suggesting for a moment that you're a lazy couch potato, it's another study that shows limited activities and interests are likely to contribute to a drop in brain performance and health.

There are limitations to the study findings that require further research; however, these findings align with a commonly used expression, 'Variety is the spice of life.' This expression was inspired by a similar line from a poem published in 1785, written by William Cowper.[20] Written over 230 years ago, this poem reminds us that we don't always have to understand science to know why something feels good for our brain. The most important thing is that it just does, and that's good enough.

There is likely a connection between your brain's electrical activity and the benefit of variety and diversity in your activities. Earlier in the book, I mentioned that your brain's neurons communicate with each other via electrical and chemical signals. These electrical signals are called brain waves and happen at different frequencies, and don't occur in isolation because different waves happen at the same time inside the brain. The five main frequencies that have been detected by scientists are gamma, beta, alpha, theta and delta, which are written here in the order of their intensity. Gamma is the fastest wave, and delta is the slowest.

We don't need to go deep into the science of brain waves, but it's useful to know that the different speeds relate to various processes inside your brain. For example, alpha waves are associated with feeling physically and mentally relaxed, while the faster beta waves are associated with focusing on a task, actively listening, and learning. Theta waves are much slower and are related to deep relaxation and daydreaming.

....

This could partially explain why variety and diversity are essential to your brain's ongoing performance.

....

The main point here is that different brain waves are associated with the various complex processing demands on your brain. The diversity and variety in your activities also mean your brain waves may be changing more regularly between high and low frequencies, which may help reduce the feeling of fatigue that can happen when we don't take a break from learning, focusing on complex tasks or problem-solving to do something else at a different pace, like a relaxing hobby or listening to music.

Maitlan Brown, a professional athlete I first worked with a few years ago, is a fabulous example of how diversity and variety can improve your life. Since we started working together, Maitlan has grown her interests to a remarkable level of diversity as a gardener, cook, golfer, designer, dog mum, cyclist and cricketer.

One thing we worked on in the early days was creating a mindset built on diverse interests, not just cricket and her design studies. Maitlan doesn't need more help from me with this mindset because she has sorted that out herself. And it's not a matter of Maitlan filling every waking moment with these activities. She also takes care of her brain in other ways, including the different strategies in this book.

While I may not have the same repertoire of activities and interests that Maitlan does, my quality of life and overall energy has been trans-formed as I introduced more variety and diversity into my life. I am no longer fixated or obsessed about work or any other 'one thing', as I now have diverse creative, professional and social interests across various areas of my life.

FRESH EXPERIENCES ARE A SOURCE OF ENERGY FOR YOUR BRAIN

One of the explanations for brain fatigue I proposed in chapter one is that your brain has had enough and can't be bothered continuing with whatever it is you're doing. Perhaps this happens because your brain predicts that the value of the task is not worth the energy required to continue doing it. Having diverse interests and activities in your life is perhaps one way you can reduce how often you feel mentally and physically fatigued. Creating fresh experiences for your brain during the day will also likely influence where you're sitting on the Brain Energy Continuum (BEC).

....

Maybe the chemistry inside you at that point in time is
no longer stimulating your brain to keep going.

....

If you're feeling fatigued and sluggish, switching your energy to doing something else can create opportunities for your brain to recover and feel energised again. Becoming more deliberate in prioritising your brain's position on the BEC is critical to becoming a Brainy Athlete. Mixing up your day with various activities, even if it's only ten minutes here and there of doing something different, will help you achieve this.

In my experience, including variety and diversity is essential for our brain's performance and wellbeing. I deliberately mix up the flow of my workshops so participants can do various activities. During a ninety-minute session on self-leadership, for instance, I usually include a brief intro, play a short video, show some simple slides, encourage whole group discussions, write and draw on a whiteboard, ask participants to complete a small group activity, ask them questions, explain concepts, and include a break to switch off from the session altogether. You can see that in the space of ninety minutes, there is a lot of diversity and variety. Have you thought about creating similar routines that blend diversity in your workplace, at home, or anywhere else? You may be limited or restricted due to your environment, time, or other people's needs; however, you may be more in control of your choices than you realise.

What about an alternative delivery style for my workshop? Say I give the participants a lecture for ninety long and torturous minutes, supported by a zillion slides, with no breaks or group discussions, and five minutes at the end for questions. I probably won't get one question because everyone in that room, including me, is tired, bored and disengaged. People start checking their phones, yawning, and some even fall asleep. This is a sure sign that their brains are fatigued, and their performance has dropped significantly. It's also a sure sign that I should get another job or change my delivery style quickly if I worked this way, which I don't.

TRACK YOUR ACTIVITIES

Exploring the diversity and variety in your activities starts with making a checklist of what you're currently doing. This requires investigating and gathering evidence on what activities you do, how often you do them, for how long, and the flow of the activities. This will give you a clear understanding of the level of diversity and variety in your actions and a benchmark for working out what may need to change, what's working, and what may be getting in the way of your brain's performance and health.

I wouldn't rely on your memory of the past few days to do this because much of the information will be flawed, biased, imagined or wrong. When your brain recalls memories, it reconstructs what happened using chemicals and electrical signals to communicate between your billions of neurons. It doesn't work like a photo or video file because your brain recreates memories whenever you think of them. This means your memories can be very different from what you've been doing for the past week.

Instead, I recommend monitoring your activity for one to two weeks and recording this in a written or electronic journal. At least one week means every day is included, and two weeks is better because it may identify fluctuations between weeks. The information I suggest you record includes the type of activity, duration, any breaks, and when you did it.

I also recommend several categories to group activities together, because having diverse interests was shown to be important for brain performance in the research considered earlier in this chapter. Grouping similar activities together helps identify whether most of your activities are related to one area of your life. For example, if you spend most of your time on activities related only to work or your sport, this may identify variety but a lack of diversity in your activities.

Once you have a clearer understanding of the level of diversity and variety in your activities, you have valuable evidence to make informed decisions about your routines and whether any adjustments or changes need to be made to prioritise your brain.

Head to my website at www.gazmills.com/brainyresources and you'll find a template that you can use to record your activity accurately. You can record how each activity you track influences a Brainy Athlete, which can help you prioritise your current activities and decide what may need to stay or go.

I have introduced this activity early in the book because you can use the information you record to help guide your understanding and decisions as you learn more about becoming a Brainy Athlete from the following chapters.

Recording your activities is a critical step to understanding what's happening now, so your decisions and actions lead you towards becoming a Brainy Athlete.

CHAPTER HIGHLIGHTS

1. A lack of variety and diversity in your life can lead to overtraining for your brain.
2. Studies have revealed that people with various diverse interests and activities showed higher brain performance than people with less diversity and variety in their lives.
3. Mixing up your day with diverse experiences helps reduce the risk of brain fatigue resulting from your brain being tired of doing the same thing for too long.
4. Simply switching regularly between diverse activities can positively impact your brain's performance.
5. Track your activities for one to two weeks to identify where you can make the most of variety and diversity in your daily life. Use the template from my website to start tracking your activities today, and use the information to help you through the rest of this book.

Chapter 4

Lead Your Lazy Brain

Keep your brain's eye on the prize

A few years ago, I was a police bodyguard for the Australian Prime Minister and other leaders around the world, who we called the 'principal.' Some of it was like what you see on TV shows or in a movie, but mostly it wasn't. Mostly, it involved standing around for hours, travelling inside cars and planes, walking between buildings and cars and planes, and completing the administration that surrounded everything we did. It was one of those jobs where you had to learn to switch on even when it was mundane and slow, which it often was. In some ways, it was a lot like playing sports.

....

I was a bodyguard for an Australian Prime Minister.

....

A few years ago, I was a bodyguard for former Australian Prime Minister John Howard. 'PM' as we called him, was a sports fanatic and went to more than a few major sports events. That was great because it meant I got to go to a few of those events, including the Rugby World Cup, Davis Cup tennis, and international cricket tests. Not a bad gig for someone who also loves sports.

I often went out with PM on his early morning walks. He was famous for these 6 am walks, and most people ask me about them when they find out what I used to do. PM usually wore his Aussie team tracksuit, and we would follow on foot and in vehicles – without wearing matching Aussie tracksuits. PM walked fast for about thirty minutes and rarely missed his morning walk. He had his routine for physical activity despite his job running the country. I think there's something in that for everybody who says they can't find any time for physical activity.

While PM's physical routine was good, his choices around where he wanted to walk presented an extra challenge for us. He had his favourite routes, and we repeated them day after day. We had a saying when I was a bodyguard: 'Routine can get you killed,' meaning if you follow the same physical movements over and over, you become predictable and make it easier for the bad guys to track you. In the case of the PM, it was routine where he went for his morning walks in Sydney and Canberra.

I don't blame the PM for his walking routine because where we walked was beautiful and a fantastic way to start the day. For example, in Sydney, we walked next to Sydney Harbour, Luna Park and Lavender Bay. The views don't get much better than that in Sydney, and if he wanted to walk that way every day, there was not much we could do about it in the absence of any specific instructions saying that he shouldn't.

FOLLOWING THE BOUNCING BALL

While there is some truth to the 'routine can get you killed' statement in certain environments, routines are also good because they establish expectations, maintain standards, promote safety and drive consistency. As a bodyguard, following agreed routines ensured everyone was working off the same script, not taking shortcuts, and not making things up on the run without letting everybody else know about it.

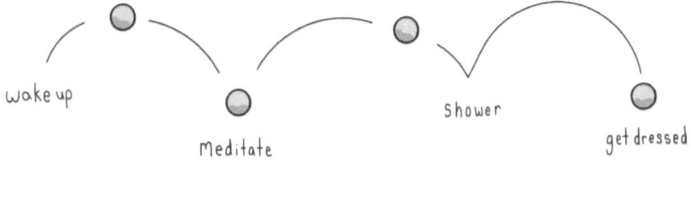

wake up · Meditate · Shower · get dressed

....

Routines are a guide for your brain to follow the bouncing ball.

....

Routines mean your brain doesn't have to work as hard because it takes out a lot of the guess work and uncertainty, which is a good thing for your brain's energy flow. It also ensures you're more consistent with your behaviours. When we repeat our routines and see we're making progress, that can motivate us to repeat them.

An example of a routine for triathletes is how they set up their cycling and running gear. One routine may be clipping their cycling shoes on their bike pedals during set up so they can get out on their bike quicker by sliding their feet into the shoes while riding. I do this, and when I stick to my practised routines, things usually go smoothly. But what about that time I was doing an Ironman 70.3 on the Sunshine Coast in Queensland? I set up for the transition in dim light because I forgot to bring a torch or my phone, which was part of my routine. I went largely by feel, including clipping my cycling shoes on my pedals. I also didn't stick to the second part of my routine, which was doing a second check of my shoes to make sure everything was set up right.

After the swim leg of the race, I removed my wetsuit, grabbed my helmet and bike, and took off on the bike course. When I tried to slip my foot into my first cycling shoe, something didn't feel right. As I pushed my toes harder into the shoe, I realised my right shoe was clipped on the left side and my left shoe on the right. A little embarrassed, but more amused, I stopped and put my shoes on the correct feet and took off again. That day is still my best 70.3 time, so maybe I need to do something amusing and a little annoying more often to perform at my best!

IS YOUR BRAIN REALLY LAZY?

Because your brain requires a lot of energy to function effectively, it has developed clever ways for streamlining many decisions and actions that conserve its energy, save you time, and free your conscious mind for more important things. In this chapter, we will look at routines and habits.

....

While I often say our brain is lazy, it really is amazingly efficient and resourceful.

....

Routines require some conscious thought because they're not automatic. Our routines tend to happen in a particular order, like your bedtime routine. Habits are automatic behaviours, and author James Clear, in his #1 bestseller book *Atomic Habits,* defines a habit as 'the small decisions you make and actions you perform every day.'[21] Clear's book is arguably the most comprehensive guide to habits in recent years, and his definition of habits is simple and (pardon the pun) very clear.

Bruce Lipton, world-renowned cell biologist and author of *The Biology of Belief,* explains that 'scientific assessments reveal that the wishes, desires, and aspirations of our creative conscious minds only control cognitive behaviour about 5% of the time.'[22] This means that ninety-five per cent of the time your subconscious mind is in charge and you behave automatically without thinking about what you're doing. Dr Lipton says your 'subconscious mind is habitual.'

Because routines involve deliberate thinking but habits don't, we can use our routines to help create habit change. You can consider your existing routines and look for opportunities to create new habits that help you be a Brainy Athlete.

We all have routines and habits that are more supportive of our athletic goals than others. Some help us, and others don't. One example is when we automatically reach for our mobile phone to scroll, surf or message as soon as we get distracted from whatever else it is we're doing. I still go for the unconscious phone grab, but I'm much better at catching myself before I become lost in time and my brain starts to drain energy.

....

A personal challenge we all face is our internal struggle between staying on track for our long-term goals and satisfying our immediate urges.

....

An example is the struggle between getting up at 5am to train versus hitting the snooze button to enjoy the cosiness of your warm bed in winter. Remember that your brain's main job is to look after your body, so in this case, it predicts that resting in bed is a better investment for your body than using energy to exercise in the cold for a race that's six weeks away. It sounds like your brain is lazy, but it's doing what it thinks is in your body's best interests. For this reason and more, try developing routines and habits to reinforce your Brainy Athlete behaviours.

Habits and routines include putting on your cycling helmet and turning the rear adjustment dial six clicks every time. Another is a cricketer facing the next ball and always tapping their bat on the ground eight times without counting because they've done it thousands of times before. Another is feeling nervous the night before a race, and automatically grabbing a bag of Oreo cookies and eating them all before your conscious brain realises you've finished the lot.

When you create new habits and routines, you're multiplying their positive effect because your brain requires less effort to follow them. Not only is your brain getting more love and care from your Brainy Athlete lifestyle, but over time your brain will use less energy as the connections in your brain drive your habits and routines to become stronger.

CREATING NEW HABITS AND ROUTINES

Creating new habits and routines doesn't necessarily mean gaining success quickly, because you need time, repetition and consistency to strengthen the connections in your brain. How quickly this happens depends on your new behaviour's complexity and commitment to learning and practising. Your new behaviours also require more cognitive resources to develop, which burns more brain energy. Even though your brain will use more energy in the short term to develop your Brainy Athlete strategies, your return on investment is worth every bit of the glucose, water, salt, and other chemicals needed.

Your environment and routines play a big part in shaping and supporting your habits, which then play a significant role in all areas of your life. If there's a habit you need to break, or a habit you want to create or continue, give yourself a nudge in the right direction through small changes to your environment and routines. The concept of nudging is attributed to the book *Nudge: Improving Decisions about Health, Wealth, and Happiness*. [23] The authors explain that 'Nudges are not mandates. Putting fruit at eye level counts as a nudge. Banning junk food does not.'

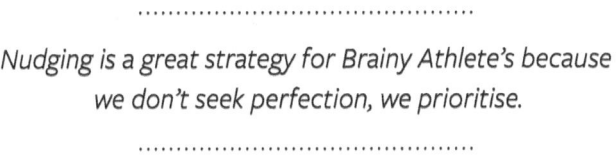

*Nudging is a great strategy for Brainy Athlete's because
we don't seek perfection, we prioritise.*

Richard Thaler, one of the book's authors, has received the Nobel Memorial Prize in Economic Sciences for his contributions to behavioural economics. Nudging can be applied to any area of your life and it's used by governments, corporations, small businesses and parents to influence decisions and behaviours.

This book will help you identify opportunities to create new habits and nudge your routines or environment so they are more brain friendly.

To explain this, I will expand on the fruit and junk food quote in the previous paragraph. This will demonstrate how you can make a small change to your existing routine and environment to stop one habit and create a new Brainy Athlete habit.

Say you have a sweet tooth, and you find yourself regularly and automatically grabbing sweet chocolate or sugar-filled cookies from the pantry when you're feeling tired and hungry. You've decided to become a Brainy Athlete, and like me, you want to restrict these sweets to a special treat you only have occasionally. You want to break this sweet habit and eat something nutritious instead, so you change your routine and environment slightly when you come home to put away the groceries.

You deliberately put sweet treats like chocolate on the top shelf, out of easy reach, instead of in the lower cupboard. You also fill a bowl, in easy reach on the kitchen bench, with fruit. Now when you're hungry and feeling peckish, it's easy to pick up an apple, but requires some conscious thought and effort to get to the sweets, so eating them is no longer automatic. You have time and space to make better choices instead of munching down a sugar-filled treat before you realise what's happening.

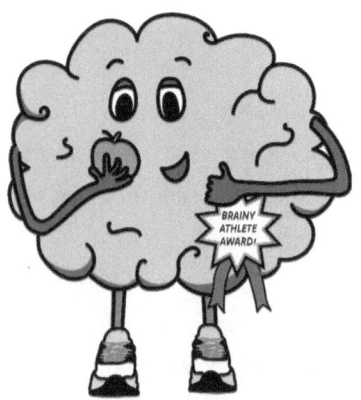

To identify what opportunities and choices you have for creating Brainy Athlete routines and environments, grab a piece of paper and a pen, then answer the following four questions about wherever you are now. You won't have all the answers, because you haven't finished the book and I've put you on the spot without any warning. But just do your best and start prioritising, not perfecting.

1. How are my environment and routines currently supporting the Brainy Athlete habits I want to keep?
2. How are my environment and routines currently supporting unhelpful habits I want to stop?
3. What changes could I make in my environment and routines to support new and existing Brainy Athlete habits?
4. What could I change in my environment or routines to help me stop any unhelpful habits?

As you work your way through this book, go back to your list to review and make any additions or changes. Understanding that your brain makes most of your decisions automatically and your routines create the environment for many of your habits is an important step to making changes to help you become a Brainy Athlete. Simply making small changes to your routines can create new habits, break old ones, and help you live more consistently closer to the right of the BEC.

CHAPTER HIGHLIGHTS

1. Routines and habits are building blocks for the behaviours of a Brainy Athlete.
2. Routines require deliberate thinking, while habits do not.
3. Small changes to routines can create new habits and break old ones.
4. Creating new routines and habits doesn't guarantee success quickly, because your brain needs time, repetition and consistency for them to become automatic.
5. Grab a pen and paper and start making your list now.

Chapter 5

When Less Is More

*Feel more alive living your life
instead of someone else's*

Sitting here writing this chapter, I just checked my email inboxes, and there are over 54,000 messages in there. Seventeen thousand are unread emails, so I'm sorry if I haven't replied to yours yet. I should get to it by 2033, but it's best you email me again to get to the top of the list. I've unsubscribed from a few, but even that takes time, which is why thousands of unopened emails exist.

One major source of my many emails is the athletic events I attend or compete at. Afterwards, I get bombarded with emails from the event organisers, sponsors and suppliers. There are offers to sign up for next year's event at a discount because I'm told demand will be high, and I don't want to miss out. They also send emails about other events they run that I also don't want to miss out on. I get offers to complete a survey and go in the draw to win cash or entry to another event.

Then there are more emails from sponsors who offer the latest and greatest products and services. There are training offers guaranteed to make me stronger, faster and fitter. There's new gear that promises to make me the coolest kid on the block or take seconds off my over-all time to beat the competition. I need to slice off more than a few seconds at the speed I go to win.

There are event emails reminding me that if I don't register for the race by a certain time, I miss out on my name being included on the official t-shirt. One of those emails told me I can't miss the t-shirt deadline because there's 'no better feeling than being able to point out your name in the list of athletes competing to all of your family and friends.'

....

While it's cool to be part of the official merchandise, I hope there are better feels from a race than my name being printed on a t-shirt.

....

These emails can quickly become the catalyst for signing up for almost every event that remotely relates to my sport. If we don't go, we miss out on the event itself and the networking and social connections that go with it. Athletes who do go enjoy the event, mixing with other ath-letes and enjoying the rich experiences. We know they do because we see it on their social media feeds, having all the fun and glory, while we can only dream of what could have been. Then we sign up for twenty events during the next two months so we don't miss out and can do more than just dream about it.

This is not that different from our life outside of sports. For example, I get regular invites to different business networking events, which are generally breakfasts or after-work meetups. An event could include a guest speaker, expert panel, or just an opportunity to socialise and build connections. These are good business and social opportunities, but also time intensive if you let it get out of hand and put your hand up for every opportunity that comes your way. But I should go to as many as I can, shouldn't I? If I don't go, I might miss out on meeting someone important to my business, or people might stop inviting me along. I'll be all on my own. That might sound dramatic, but we can fall into the trap of going to almost every function when we worry more about what we might miss if we *don't* go than what we might gain if we *do*. I know people who go to almost everything, and I don't know when they find time to work or sleep.

We also find ourselves fully booked and even overcommitting to our social lives. We say yes to everything because we don't want to miss out, or we worry about what people might think if we say no to going. While writing this, it's three weeks until the end of 2022. This time of the year in Australia is especially busy with work lunches, after-work drinks, parties, school holidays, visiting family and friends, trips to the beach, and my favourite sports event, the Boxing Day Test at the Melbourne Cricket Ground. Many athletes, including me, are still working, training, competing, and taking care of all the personal stuff in our lives.

....

There will always be only twenty-four hours in a day,
and we can't be everywhere at once.

....

When we overly worry that we're missing out on something or someone, our brain can struggle to rest and recover from our response to the chemicals cascading around our brain and body. When our fear of missing out becomes a problem, and we make poor choices, this is a barrier to making good choices that are necessary to become a Brainy Athlete.

WHAT ARE YOU MISSING?

The fear of missing out, or FOMO as it's commonly known, can be described as 'the uneasy and sometimes all-consuming feeling that you're missing out – that your peers are doing, in the know about, or in possession of more or something better than you.' [24]

An unhealthy obsession with FOMO will not help you be a Brainy Athlete. For example, a recent article published in *PsychCentral* explains that FOMO can 'impact your sleep and eating habits' and lead to 'fatigue, headaches, lack of motivation, performance issues at work or school, and burnout.' [25] This means FOMO has been found to negatively impact at least two fundamental Brainy Athlete strategies in this book, which are sleep and fuel.

....

FOMO's explosion from social media is widely reported; however, the FOMO concept is not new.

....

In fact, we can trace the FOMO factor back to 1913 when American cartoonist Arthur R. 'Pop' Momand created the phrase, 'Keeping up with the Joneses,' for his comic strip. This phrase describes an obsession to keep pace with what your neighbours have or are doing. For example, if your neighbour buys a new car or puts in a swimming pool, you feel you must do it too; otherwise, you risk falling behind them on the social ladder. You can imagine how this belief can lead to poor choices driven by excessive worry, embarrassment, ego, and our need to fit in or belong.

Clinical psychologist and Harvard Medical School instructor Natalie Christine Dattilo PhD, explained to Forbes Health online in 2022 that FOMO 'is closely related to the fear of social exclusion or ostracism, which existed long before social media.' [26]

For example, if you feel mentally exhausted today, but some friends have a social dinner tonight, you may force yourself to go. After all, you worry your mates will think less of you or talk about you because you're not there. You may worry that this social group could shun you, which would be horrible. FOMO overrides your brain and body's desperate need to rest and recover, so you'll pay the price mentally and physically tomorrow, and perhaps longer than that. You struggle to get out of bed the next day for an important training session and put in a half-baked effort that throws your whole training week out. All for a dinner you felt too tired to go to, but FOMO got the better of you. In the end you didn't really enjoy yourself and people were asking you all night what was wrong because you weren't your usual self.

....

Not only can we fear missing out on something now, but we also worry that others might exclude us in the future.

....

Another example is turning up to training with your club, and someone who is a friendly rival has a new bike with all the bling that allegedly makes it super light and lightning quick. You look at your bike, which might be only two years older and 500 g heavier, but the weight of disappointment and jealousy on your shoulders feels like a tonne. Two minutes ago, you loved your bike. Now it's an embarrassment.

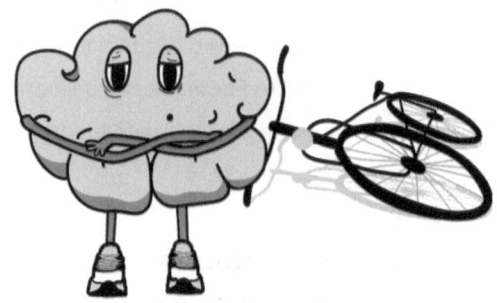

Social media has made it much easier to check out what our ever-expanding virtual networks are thinking, saying, doing and buying. This social information flow is 24/7 and endless, which means that you can spend hours reading posts, watching videos, clicking links and checking out people's profiles any time of the day. We may respond by posting our own photos and videos to keep up with the Joneses, which is time-consuming, mentally draining, and contributes to the never-ending FOMO problem.

WHEN COMPARISONS BECOME AN OBSESSION

Unfortunately, when comparing our life to what's happening on social media becomes an obsession, it also becomes a barrier to being a Brainy Athlete. We look at what everyone else is doing in our online networks and form judgements about ourselves, where we sit on the social ladder, and if we're missing out on what other people are experiencing. We see people at races or events that we're not attending. We look at videos of athletes we know on podiums, smiling with other athletes at coffee shops, enjoying the finish line feel we all love, and anything else that looks a lot more fabulous than what we're doing. Sometimes it only takes one post to send us rushing down the FOMO pathway.

Another FOMO example could be comparing my athletic ability and lifestyle to a full-time, world-class athlete on Instagram who is twenty-five years younger and has a mansion in Monaco and a private helicopter. It's okay to compare because that's what our brain does all the time, but if I start worrying that my life is rubbish because my benchmark is this athlete, that's a serious problem.

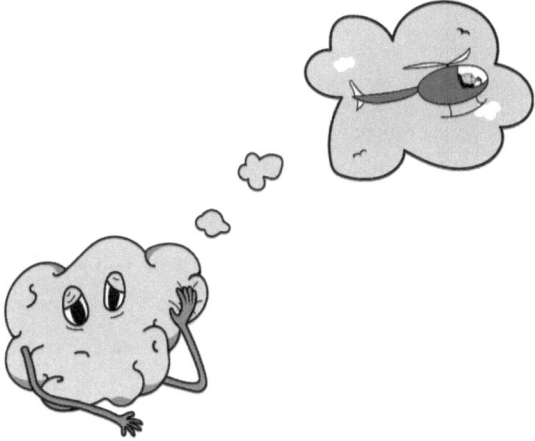

Comparisons will happen all the time, but how we interpret them will determine how our brain and body respond. This will guide your sense of belonging. For athletes, we benchmark ourselves against other athletes and where we think we fit in the sporting community. It doesn't matter if your assessment is true, because it depends on how your brain interprets and processes the chemicals that come from your comparisons that is the source of your motivation, distraction, exhaustion, excitement, disappointment, happiness, worry, love, fear or regret. For example, if your heart rate increases in response to a cool video someone posted from a race you're not at, your brain can interpret your heart rate change as motivation or FOMO. It's the same chemical experience, but your brain determines your thoughts.

A Forbes Health article describes symptoms of FOMO, including:

- overscheduling (trying to be everywhere at all times),
- feeling mentally exhausted from social media,
- feeling physically tired,
- difficulty concentrating, and
- having trouble sleeping. [26]

These symptoms scream brain fatigue. Your sleep, screentime, and how you fuel your brain are just three strategies in this book that are impacted directly by FOMO. If you regularly overload your schedule with commitments, you risk tiring your brain out and the flow-on effects of a disrupted sleeping pattern, which becomes a loop that magnifies the problem. This cycle provides minimal opportunity for your brain to rest and recover. To make matters worse, FOMO can also cause physical fatigue, which will also impact your athletic performance.

FOMO is fed by habitual behaviours such as feeling a strong urge to look at your phone as soon as you receive a notification. An example is when your phone beeps while you're talking to someone, and before you know it, you've pulled your phone out of your pocket to check it. Alternatively, you may become so distracted by the urge to check your phone that you tune out from your conversation and don't hear a word the other person is saying.

If FOMO is a problem for you, the strategies in this book will help you get rid of its tight grip. Vice versa, when FOMO is no longer a problem, you will discover more opportunities to live the Brainy Athlete strategies. It's a win-win.

FEEL MORE ALIVE LIVING YOUR LIFE

I mentioned earlier that a loop can be created when FOMO feeds unhelpful thoughts and behaviours, making your FOMO experience more intense. Your key is to break this cycle, and you can do this by applying the Brainy Athlete strategies.

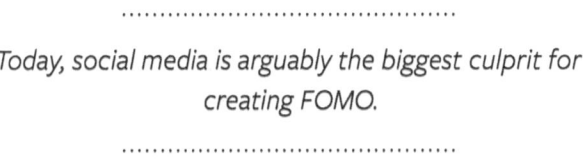

Today, social media is arguably the biggest culprit for creating FOMO.

If you need to change your habits to begin reducing the amount of time you spend on social media, there are several things you can immediately do. *Chapter 9: Streamline your Screentime* provides some tips and tricks to help you reduce your time on your phone and other digital devices. The chapter also details the science behind our strong attachment to our smart devices and how we can break the cycle.

There are Brainy Athlete strategies that will enrich your life in ways that will prevent you from feeling like you're missing out on too much. For example, chapter four is all about bringing variety and fresh experiences into your life, which means you can worry less about what others are doing or what they have. People may experience FOMO from seeing what you get up to, but for their sake, I hope they get on with enriching their own lives instead.

While other Brainy Athlete strategies will help reduce your FOMO, the last one I'll single out here is *Chapter 10: Be Less Mind-full*. Mindfulness is a superpower that broke the grip FOMO, and other debilitating thoughts, had over me for decades. Becoming more in tune with my immediate surroundings and having greater control over my brain's attention has significantly improved my ability to challenge negative thoughts, appreciate what exists today, and have more positive and rewarding relationships with the physical world around me. As a result, I am a lot more grateful for my life and the experiences I am having now. I rarely live in the past, or future, or long for a life someone else has. You can experience this and more as you loosen the grip FOMO has over you. When that happens, you have more time to live your life as a Brainy Athlete.

CHAPTER HIGHLIGHTS

1. FOMO is being obsessed with comparisons, connections and a sense of belonging.
2. FOMO can create problems that reduce your athletic performance.
3. Social media amplified the problem, but FOMO was happening long before it came along.
4. Strategies in this book will help you break the FOMO cycle.
5. As you break the FOMO cycle, you become more grateful for what you have, who you are, and what you've done.

Chapter 6

Snoozing Isn't Losing

Show up stronger tomorrow by prioritising how you finish today

In September 2022, the best cyclists in the world came to Wollongong in Australia for the UCI World Championships. I've fallen in love with cycling in recent years as a spectator and an athlete. I love watching the Tour de France and other professional races on TV. The European races are usually on late at night in Australia, so our routine at home is to either get up early and watch the previous day's highlights before work or watch them that evening.

You can imagine I was excited that the world's best would be racing only three hours from where I live. I had never experienced that before, and as it turned out, I made it to the men's road race on the Sunday. Dave, a mate of mine, loves his cycling too and joined me for the early drive to Wollongong, with the compulsory coffee stop on the way. We both had a sausage roll from the bakery too, which we knew would help with the big day of spectating ahead of us. That sounds ridiculous, but after being an injured spectator at a couple of triathlons my wife and friends were competing at, I know it's hard work watching from the sidelines for hours.

While Dave and I were making our way to Wollongong, we chatted a lot, mostly about sports. Dave also coaches athletes and knows a lot about things I'm interested in. We talked about this book I was writing, and I threw a few ideas about chapters and concepts at him for feedback. Thanks for your free expert advice, Dave. I owe you one!

When I told Dave I included this chapter on sleep and its relationship to brain fatigue for athletes, he told me about an experience he had coaching one of his former athletes. I know this athlete too and out of respect for them and their privacy, I'll keep any personal stuff out of the story. Let's call this athlete Gabby.

WHEN FATIGUE CATCHES UP WITH YOU

Gabby had big goals as an endurance athlete and put her heart and soul into training. Gabby's endurance increased significantly while working with Dave, but there was a period when Gabby's performance plateaued and she felt fatigued a lot of the time. This impacted how hard and long she could train, and she couldn't understand why she felt so drained. And because she couldn't get the most out of her training sessions, she did some extra training that only worsened her fatigue.

Dave did what good coaches do: asked Gabby a bunch of questions to get to the root cause of her slump. As it turned out, Gabby had a problem that would make any of us feel mentally and physically exhausted. She was having less than six hours of sleep a night. No wonder Gabby was so fatigued, and her athletic performance was suffering. I'm impressed that Gabby could perform to the level she did, even though it was below her best.

Ironically, at the men's road race in Wollongong, there was a notable withdrawal as the result of a poor night of sleep. Dutch cyclist Mathieu van der Poel, one of the pre-race favourites, abandoned the race an hour after starting because he was exhausted, which is hard to imagine for a rider of his quality and experience. Van der Poel's performance was way below his best because of an incident at his hotel the night before, which caused him to have a shocking sleep. Even the best athletes in the world are not immune to the effects a poor sleep has on their performance.

OUR CHOICES CREATE SLEEP PROBLEMS

'You snooze, you lose' is defined in the Cambridge Dictionary as 'if you do not pay attention and do something quickly, someone else will do it instead of you.' While there is some truth to this statement for seizing opportunities or an advantage, it is unhelpful if you apply it to the relationship between your brain's need to sleep and optimising your athletic performance.

....

Your brain needs quality sleep, and many people don't appear to be getting that.

....

While there are various reasons why people don't get enough sleep, the statistics are worrying. Research by Deloitte for the Sleep Health Foundation in 2017 estimates that nearly forty per cent, or 7.4 million, adult Australians 'experience some form of inadequate sleep.' Sleep disorders and other health problems affecting sleep account for just under half this estimate, while 3.8 million people 'routinely fail to get enough sleep, often suffering side effects of sleep deprivation.' [27]

In 2019, Professor Peter Eastwood, Director of the University of Western Australia Centre for Sleep Science, said many people were experiencing insufficient sleep due to 'poor sleep hygiene, poor sleep measures and lifestyle problems.' [28] Again, these are worrying signs that are even more troubling considering many people's choices are leading to poor sleeping habits. Choices that affect our sleep are the focus of this chapter. Please keep in mind that this chapter does not address any sleeping disorders or other health conditions that may be affecting your sleep or anyone else's. Please chat to a health professional if you're concerned about any health condition you may have.

The Australian Sleep Health Foundation recommends seven to nine hours of sleep for adults aged between eighteen and sixty-four. Less than six hours or more than eleven hours are not recommended. [29] Around seven and a half hours a night is usually enough for me to feel well rested and ready to go; however, it will also depend on what I did the previous day and if I stuck to my bedtime routine.

You may have met people who say they can function effectively on six hours of sleep or less every night. We hate those people because one six-hour sleep can ruin our whole week. Researchers have identified mutant genes that may be the reason some people feel fully rested after less than six hours of sleep. [30] However, study sample sizes are small, and there's no long-term data, so we can't be sure about the effects on the brain and body of people who have a mutant gene.

Regardless, the mutant gene seems very rare, and researchers have estimated that only three percent of the population has it. [30] I have no idea if I have the mutant gene or not, but I do know that, like millions of other Australians, I need more than six hours of sleep to be anywhere near my best and, based on Gabby's sleep experiences, she does too.

Another potential problem for your brain's performance comes from a study that suggests if you are totally sleep deprived for one night, it takes more than two nights of quality sleep to fully restore your memory's performance. [31] While it's unlikely you would deliberately pull an all-nighter close to a race, this finding suggests that after having a crappy night's sleep, your brain's performance could be impaired for longer than expected or hoped. This could disrupt or derail your race preparation and outcome.

INSUFFICIENT SLEEP SYNDROME

Your brain goes through various stages of activity while you sleep. These include rapid eye movement and deep sleep stages that make up 'four to six sleep cycles that range from 70 to 120 minutes each.' Each stage impacts your brain differently because 'different chemicals in the brain become activated or deactivated to coordinate rest and recovery.' [32] When you miss cycles due to poor quality sleep, your brain misses out on some of the chemical processes it needs to rest and recover.

....

*Insufficient sleep results in your brain missing
opportunities to flush out toxins, process memories,
repair cells and reinforce your learning.*

....

There's a name that describes the condition of not getting enough
sleep – insufficient sleep syndrome (ISS). The American Academy of
Sleep Medicine says that people with ISS may 'have concentration and
attention problems, lowered energy level, reduced alertness, distracti-
bility, irritability or fatigue.' [33] Any one of these will cost you something
as an athlete, and more than one of these symptoms can be disastrous
for your performance.

Another reason to prioritise your sleep is 'brain functions associated
with pain inhibition have also been shown to be reduced' when fatigue
is caused by sleep loss.' [34] [35] This means that when your brain is well
rested, you should have a higher tolerance for the feelings of discomfort that come from pushing yourself at training and in competition. If
you want to improve your fitness and performance, it's inevitable that
you will experience discomfort, and if you can suffer more for longer,
your results should improve.

Brain researchers have explored the effect sleep deprivation has on
our cognitive flexibility, which is our ability to adapt our thought processes to changing circumstances. Unexpected and surprising things
can happen to athletes when competing, which tests their ability to
adjust the existing strategy to the unfolding circumstances. For example,
I've had mechanical issues and injuries and made rookie errors during
triathlon races that required cognitive flexibility to overcome the issue

or just make the best of a situation. Our mental ability to recognise changing circumstances, identify solutions, and execute them while continuing to compete is critical for our performance outcome.

One study on brain performance showed that the brain's ability to adjust to changing circumstances successfully is 'more negatively affected' by sleep deprivation than an unchanging situation.[36] From an athlete's perspective, this means that a pre-planned strategy is less affected by sleep-induced fatigue than a strategy we need to adjust in response to what's unfolding during competition or at training. This makes sense when we consider that our brain works harder and uses more energy when it's experiencing something new, like changing circumstances during a race. In contrast, an already sleep-fatigued brain will find it easier to stick to the original race plan and follow the bouncing ball than try to process something new.

A well-rested brain puts you in the best position to be an agile athlete who can respond effectively and quickly to changes in the game or race.

GOOD SLEEP COMES FROM YOUR ROUTINES

Sleep disorders aside, one of the simplest changes we can make in our lives that delivers broad benefits is to prioritise our sleep. When we remove the barriers preventing us from getting a good night's sleep, we let neurobiology do its work for our brain while we enjoy slumberland.

The effects we're seeking with our sleep routine won't always happen because we all have nights when we have a less than ideal, or even terrible, sleep. This can be caused by staying up late to meet an urgent work deadline, leaving an assignment to the last minute (again), watching live sports on TV in a different time zone, or partying until the early hours of the morning. Other times excessive worrying about things that have happened or might happen can cause us to have a restless sleep.

....

The goal is to establish good routines that prepare you for a good night's sleep and help you get back to sleep if you wake up in the middle of the night.

....

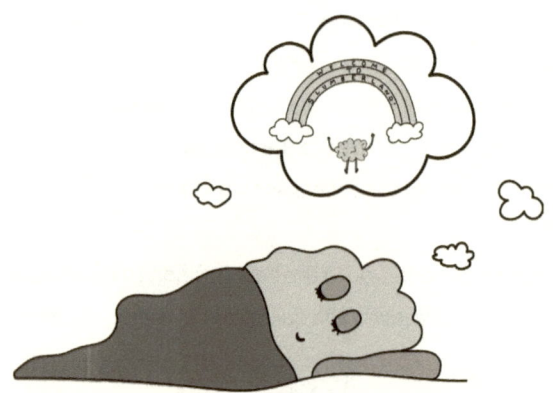

I have changed a few of my sleeping habits over recent years, which has significantly improved my sleep quality and energy levels. As a result, I consistently experience less fatigue while awake, think with more clarity and creativity, am less moody or emotionally unpredictable, feel healthier, and can focus for longer. I have also noticed my self-awareness is stronger because I am more in tune with what I'm experiencing inside and what's happening around me. I'll now share with you some of the most effective strategies that have helped me.

I seldom use my computer or smartphone once I'm in bed before sleep. Instead, I grab a pen and my latest Sudoku puzzle book, and get solving. If I solve the puzzle, it's a sweet little win to end the day and I go to sleep with a smile. If I don't solve it, that means my brain is ready to sleep, or I picked a hard puzzle – maybe a bit of both, but I still go to sleep with a smile.

I sometimes put in my AirPods and listen to some soothing music if I need something a bit extra to wind down in bed. You can try this to help quiet your active brain, noisy neighbours or loud traffic. You can also get apps that have timed playlists and soothing sounds. This is useful if you're worried your own music library might turn to heavy metal and frighten you to near death in the middle of the night.

I sleep with a wearable health tracker device that measures my sleep quality. While I'm sleeping, it monitors my sleep cycles, heart rate, temperature, and various other body signals. In the morning, I download the data onto a phone app, and it gives me a sleep and readiness score. Over time this has helped nudge my sleeping routine to help me go to bed earlier, get up earlier, and in return have better quality sleep. One thing it educated me on is my deep sleep – I need to go to bed earlier than I used to for deep sleep, which makes sense because most deep sleep happens in the first half of the night.

When I feel tired during the day because something has affected my brain's energy levels, I have been known to have a quick nap. Around thirty minutes is a good amount of time for me to feel refreshed from a light sleep and not groggy from a deeper sleep. I had an executive job a few years ago, and our staff carpark was across the road. If my brain felt so fatigued that I found it hard to function at work, I would sometimes take a quick nap in my car during my lunch break.

....

*A nap would give my brain a quick recharge so that I
could show up mentally for the afternoon and not fall
asleep at my desk, which was useful as a short-term fix.*

....

One scientific study looked at the effect of a ninety-minute nap on sleep-deprived participants, and discovered that their recovery sleep 'demonstrated the ability to restore learning ability' to 'performance levels that were not significantly different from those' experienced after a night of restful sleep. [37] While this study was small and I'm not suggesting you sacrifice quality overnight sleep by having quick power naps during the day, your brain may benefit from a short nap when you're feeling fatigued.

I used to need naps a lot more when I didn't prioritise my brain like I do now as a Brainy Athlete. Back when I was having a lot more naps, the problem could have been related to my sleeping patterns, not hydrating enough, not eating the right foods or fuelling properly after a training session, not giving my brain breaks from the computer, or rushing between meetings.

I go to bed by 10 pm most nights, or earlier if I'm tired, and I get up around 5:30 am during the week and rarely sleep past 6 am on the weekends. Most mornings I feel well rested and energised, and more time awake in the morning means I don't have to rush like a bullet train to get to where I need to be that day, whether that's out for a training ride or going to work. I never used to be an early morning person and often stayed up late, but I was able to change my sleep pattern over time by being consistent with my routine.

Another tip is to keep the lights dimmed or use lamps at night to signal your brain's biological clock to release more melatonin to help make you sleepy. It's one way to save on your power bills too. Light has the opposite effect of helping you sleep; it reduces melatonin to wake you up. That's a good reason to seek some sunlight or bright lighting when you wake up.

Research has identified that the optimal temperature for sleeping is around 18 °C or 65 °F, but this can vary a few degrees between people. If your room is too hot, this can lead to dehydration, affect your recovery, and leave you feeling fatigued the next day. Although a cooler-than-ideal bedroom can cause some disruption to your REM sleep cycle, it's less damaging to your sleep quality than a hot room. [38]

Now that you understand more about quality sleep and ways you can improve your sleep, it may be time to review and improve your sleeping environment and bedtime routine. You can do this by adding to the list you started in *Chapter 4: Lead Your Lazy Brain*. Getting a good night's sleep is not a luxury, but a necessity to be a Brainy Athlete.

CHAPTER HIGHLIGHTS

1. Prioritise your sleep quality and bed routine to help you become a Brainy Athlete.
2. If you're concerned that a sleep disorder or another health problem may affect your sleep quality, please seek medical advice.
3. Your sleep greatly influences concentration, attention, energy, wellbeing and mood.
4. Improving your sleep routine and environment is one of the most effective ways to experience broad benefits for your brain.
5. If you want to show up as your best self tomorrow, you must finish today with a good night's sleep.

Chapter 7

Fuel Your Brain

Eat and drink to start, and stay sharp

Every Ironman triathlete I have spoken to shares similar experiences to me when they recall knowing the finish line is just around the corner, or being on the red carpet and seeing it ahead of them. Knowing you're that close to the end gives you an instant boost of energy to finish off what has been a long, tough, painful day at the office.

You can hear the music pumping, fans cheering, and the race announcer's voice as they call out the names of the Ironman finishers ahead of you. I was extra lucky that Mike Reilly, the most famous voice in Ironman, was on the microphone to call my name as I finished my first Ironman at Port Macquarie, Australia, in 2018. I lapped up the energy, excitement and food in the recovery tent surrounded by dozens of exhausted, sweaty and remarkable athletes, all with newsworthy stories to share about their experiences.

I enjoyed this experience not only because I trained hard for it but also because I had a nutrition plan and stuck to it. As athletes, we know that how we choose to fuel our bodies significantly impacts our performances in training and competition. An extreme and dangerous example of what happens when we get our fuelling wrong is bonking, when you hit the wall because your energy tank is empty. Bonking can also mean something else, but that's a different discussion! If you haven't experienced bonking before, imagine your body has turned to jelly, and every new movement becomes a monumental effort because you've depleted your energy reserves.

At the 1997 Ironman World Championships in Hawaii, two elite triathletes had a memorable finish to their race, crossing the line only metres apart. It was a race finish very different from anything I've experienced, and I'm guessing that's true for most athletes. Sian Welch and Wendy Ingraham only had a few hundred metres to finish after swimming, biking, and running for 226 kilometres, or 146 miles, when something disturbing happened.

Author Tim Moria describes the finish in *Triathlon Today* like this, 'A few hundred metres before the finish, things went completely wrong, and both ladies lost control of their bodies. And, if you think you've seen the worst of it, wait until the last thirty metres. With every step they take, they collapse, try to get back on their feet, but fall down again. In the end, they crawl across the finish line, finishing fourth and fifth, respectively.' [39]

Ingraham spoke of her experience in an online article published in *Outside* and written by Bethany Mavis. She said, 'I lost my salt tablets somewhere around mile six on the run. My body started to cramp from my toes moving up to my back. It was very painful with each step.' [40] A virus reportedly led to Sian throwing up during the bike leg, leading to fuelling issues of her own. Both athletes recovered, but it's a great example of fuel's critical impact on our performance and health. If you hit the wall in training or a race and run out of energy, there's no coming back until you've rested, refuelled and recovered.

It's no different for our brain, yet people miss breakfast, make poor choices, skip meals, don't drink enough water, and wonder why their brain feels like mush and wants to sleep. What you eat or drink and how often you fuel up will impact how well your brain shows up and continues to perform.

YOUR BRAIN'S FAVOURITE BUFFET

Your brain consumes more energy than any other body part; its favourite buffet includes glucose, water, salt, fats and other chemicals. Your brain also needs oxygen to survive. Glucose comes from the carbohydrates you consume, and salt can be taken in various ways, including tablets, when you're training and racing. Your body breaks down carbohydrates into sugars, including the glucose that your brain uses for energy.

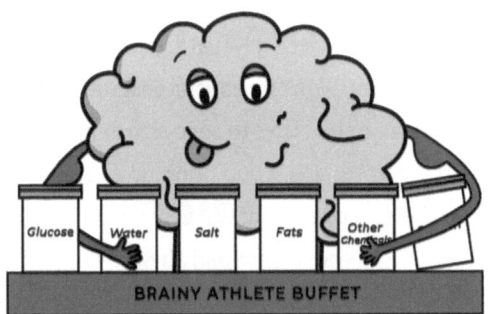

We follow a nutrition plan while training, racing and competing because as our body uses energy, we need to replenish the stocks so we can keep performing closer to our best. This is critical during endurance events where you may be on the go for hours and even days. Your body does not have unlimited energy available, so you must take more fuel in as you go, which is no different for your brain.

....

You must respect your brain's nutrition plan in the same way as your body if you expect it to perform, be healthy, and not 'bonk' when you need it.

....

A research paper by Professor Romain Meeusen, PhD, on athlete health, explains that 'fatigue during exercise can reside in the brain,' and what's happening only in your brain can influence your 'sensation of fatigue and thus potentially affect performance.' [41] Professor Meeusen says that fuelling your brain properly may determine how much your performance is affected by brain fatigue.

What you eat and drink influences what you do and how well you do it, for better or worse. Your brain is the command-and-control centre for your body, so if you don't effectively fuel it, your decisions and actions will be impaired, and you won't be at your best mentally or physically. Your brain uses various chemicals to send signals inside and between your 100 billion neurons, and if you don't take on fuel to replenish them and help their recovery, you will experience brain fatigue and feel low on energy while your mental and physical performance suffers.

I'm not here to assess or judge your nutrition choices or rate the pros and cons of the carnivore, vegan, vegetarian, keto, paleo, or any other diet against each other. I'm not a nutritionist who can tell you what you should eat, but I offer insight into how important fuelling your brain is and some helpful tips.

I encourage you to research and learn from educated professionals to make informed decisions about fuelling your brain and body rather than relying on slick advertising or articles, word of mouth or a sponsored post that promises fast and amazing results. In an information-dense market with so many choices, companies appeal to your brain's desires and fears around performance, fitness, health, body image and self-esteem. Some have your brain's best interest at heart. Others are more interested in your credit card details.

As an athlete, you likely consume a lot of fast-working sugar and caffeine in the form of supplements like gels, bars, drink mixes or homemade foods. When you're smashing it on the track or field and need to maintain your energy, get a quick boost and reduce the rate of fatigue setting in, you need something that works rapidly and effectively. You don't have time for your fuel to digest for two hours before it gives you the energy you need NOW. You will be done well before it kicks in, and so will your training session or race.

I will often use caffeine as a brain boost in races and for my harder training efforts. When I'm not training, I will have a sugar-free energy drink or an extra coffee when my brain feels tired and I need to quickly increase my alertness and focus. I can handle caffeine pretty well, and it doesn't mess with my sleep, but I know a few people who would be awake all night with tremors if they did this.

I tend to avoid sugary treats like soft drinks and lollies that give me a blood sugar spike because although they may help in the short term,

I'm aware I'll pay the price later. When I consume sugary foods and drinks, my blood sugar levels will be up and down like a yo-yo before I crash and burn. If I have downtime after a race, it may be okay to cheat a little, but if I'm working, I can't afford to crash and burn by nodding off at my desk or at the front of a training room. My brain's fuel needs to be more sustainable, smooth and consistent, so I can be too.

THE HANGRY ATHLETE

You can become hangry when you don't feed your brain enough glucose. Hangry combines the words hungry and angry and is defined in the Oxford Dictionary as 'bad-tempered or irritable as a result of hunger.' It was only added to the Oxford Dictionary in 2018, but Oxford says the word's first known use was in 1956.

....

Hanger can send even the most timid and most docile person into a rage.

....

Anger isn't the only possible reaction to being hangry. It can also result in tiredness, impatience, hostility and brain fog. Researchers from the Psychology and Neuroscience Department at the University of North Carolina suggest your hunger can be the catalyst for your emotions getting out of control. They say, 'feeling hungry can turn up the dial on lots of emotions such as anger, stress or disgust.' [42] [43]

When we skip meals, the glucose level in our blood drops, and according to gastroenterologist Dr Christine Lee, when your 'blood sugar gets too low, it triggers a cascade of hormones, including cortisol and adrenaline. These hormones are released into your bloodstream to raise and rebalance your blood sugar.' [44] These same hormones are released in response to a stressful event or something you perceive as a threat to you, priming your brain and body to survive.

....

Dr Lee explains that 'low blood sugar may interfere with higher brain functions.' This means your ability to think clearly, confidently or calmly in response to pressure may diminish.

....

Being hangry can also damage our relationships, which isn't a good thing when we usually rely on the support of our families, other athletes, coaches, supporters, officials, sponsors and volunteers to help us achieve our athletic goals. Researchers studied the link between low blood sugar levels and aggression over a 21-day study of 107 married couples. The study is called 'Low glucose relates to greater aggression in married couples,' which gives you an idea of what they were trying to understand. [45]

Every night for three weeks, each couple completed two activities to measure how upset they were with their spouse that day and the level of aggression they felt towards each other.

The first activity involved sticking pins into a voodoo doll that represented their spouse. This measured how upset they were with their spouse. The more pins they stuck in the doll, the more upset they were with their spouse.

The second activity involved having the power to blast loud and annoying sounds through the headphones their spouse was wearing. This measured their level of aggression towards their spouse. The louder and longer the sounds they chose to blast through the headphones, the stronger their level of aggression was towards their spouse.

The researchers discovered that participants 'who had lower glucose levels stuck more pins into the voodoo doll and blasted their spouse with louder and longer noise blasts.' The study didn't mention how many relationships survived the experiment, but it can be reasoned that how well we process information to make better decisions is heavily reliant on how effectively fuelled our brains are.

SUFFERING THE CONSEQUENCES

If you don't feed your brain what it needs before it's needed, it will weaken your brain's ability to process and interpret information to make good decisions. Your athletic performance can suffer in ways that include:

- reduced concentration, attention and focus,
- poor coordination and decisions that result in injury to you and others,
- increased risk of mistakes, poor judgement, errors, and
- a short fuse or inability to be reasoned with by others.

If you skip meals, your brain misses out on essential vitamins, minerals and chemicals needed to function well. If you train in the morning and don't fuel properly, it's not only your muscles missing out on the supplies needed to recover and recharge. Conversely, if you work through the day and don't fuel your brain properly, you will suffer the consequences at training and miss out on making the most of the session.

....

Fuelling your body includes hydration, not just food. Dehydration is a recipe for disaster when your brain is involved.

....

Water is estimated to account for well over half your brain's mass and is essential for your neurons to function properly. Brain scans show that our brains work harder than normal when dehydrated. An analysis of thirty-three independent studies found dehydration is more likely to impair 'high-order cognitive processing (involving attention and executive function) and motor coordination' than 'lower-order mental processing (e.g., simple reaction time).' The level of impairment was particularly noticeable when dehydration led to more than a two per cent drop in body mass.' [46]

Dehydration can harm your health, while good hydration improves sleep quality and mood. Excessive sweating caused by exercise, hot environments and other physical activity may require more hydration than normal. This should not only stand out as important for you as an athlete, but it should also register as vital to your overall success and health in life.

FUELLING YOUR BRAIN TO STAY IN THE GAME

Easy first steps to fuelling your brain are to eat healthily, drink water and not skip meals throughout the day. I know some people who regularly skip breakfast or eat very little. Unsurprisingly, they lack energy, get sleepy, become irritable, and can't think clearly. You've likely heard breakfast is the most important meal of the day and I believe this to be true. While it can be hard to make sense of all the different diets and nutrition recommendations we are constantly fed, a wholesome breakfast to kick start my day is a no brainer for me. It's called breakfast because you're breaking the fasting cycle you've had while you've been asleep for, hopefully, seven to nine quality hours.

....

Prioritise your brain by not skipping meals or leaving big gaps between fuelling up because you're too busy to eat or you forget.

....

We all get busy, so it's easy to forget things like eating and drinking or say you'll get to it later. Later is too late if you become grumpy, irrational, indecisive, or an unbearable pain to other people. It's also too late to play catch up with your fuel needs if you only remember you haven't eaten for hours or drunk enough fluids as you put on your activewear. You may still do the session, but you will do it well below what you could have done if you had fuelled your brain properly.

I am not a nutritionist, dietician, or any kind of food expert beyond knowing what I enjoy eating and drinking. However, there is significant

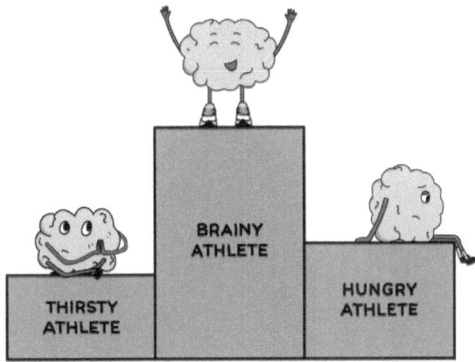

research that provides strong evidence for foods that support our brain's functioning, performance and health.

Numerous studies have identified various foods that help provide the antioxidants, vitamins and other nutrients your brain needs to optimise its performance and health. [47 48 49 50 51 52 53]

Brain-friendly foods include:

- Leafy greens
- Fatty fish
- Caffeine - coffee and green tea
- Turmeric
- Fermented foods
- Beetroot
- Broccoli
- Eggs
- Nuts, particularly walnuts
- Berries, particularly blueberries
- Numerous fruits, including oranges, apples, grapes
- Dark chocolate with >70% cocoa

- Whole grains
- Avocado
- Turkey, chicken
- Extra virgin olive oil

The benefits from eating these and other brain-boosting foods can include:

- Reducing inflammation in the brain that can impair brain function
- Promoting neurogenesis – production of new brain cells
- Defending against free radicals that can damage neurons
- Helping protect against cognitive decline and age-related memory loss
- Preventing stress-associated nerve damage

I am providing this information only as a guide on what the science says because there are other considerations that are beyond my understanding and expertise, including your specific needs and any food allergies or other risks that may exist for you. Please consult a medical or health professional for your specific nutritional and dietary needs.

Getting your nutrition right during training or competition is essential to perform at your athletic best. To be a Brainy Athlete, consider your nutritional needs in all areas of your life.

CHAPTER HIGHLIGHTS

1. Your brain consumes more energy than any other part of your body. You must feed it or you will suffer mentally and physically.

2. Just like your body, your brain needs a healthy and balanced nutrition plan to perform well, recover and remain healthy.

3. Nutrition includes drinking enough fluids, which will fluctuate depending on what you're doing or the temperature. Dehydration can harm you, while good hydration improves sleep and mood.

4. Do your research and learn from educated professionals to make informed decisions about fuelling your brain and body rather than just relying on slick advertising, word of mouth or a sponsored post that promises fast and amazing results.

5. When we skip meals, the glucose level in our blood drops and this may interfere with our higher brain function. You can get hangry – and nobody wants to be on the end of that.

Chapter 8

Nature Breaks

Take breaks in the wild to relax your brain

I love cycling outside and would choose it over my stationary trainer any day of the week. Riding my stationary bike while connected to a Bluetooth trainer indoors is handy if the weather is dangerous or if I'm really pressed for time, but I don't enjoy it as much as training outside. Some days, stationary cycling drives me crazy, and I can't wait to get off. I suppose it's one way to train my mind to be stronger and endure the suffering!

Australia is home to me, and it's legendary for its natural and diverse ecosystems. We have deserts, tropical forests, mountains, beaches, ocean reefs, national parks, wetlands and waterways scattered across the country. Whether nature was created by a god, the big bang, or something else doesn't really matter because it's here for us to appreciate and enjoy.

Our cities and urban areas also have plenty of green spaces we know were created by people and machines. These spaces include parks, sports fields, gardens, shrubberies outside buildings, communal sanctuaries on rooftops, arboretums, and nature strips between buildings and streets. Some lakes and oceans create beautiful blue spaces too.

Australia also has many cool, exotic and beautiful animals. Contrary to what many people may have heard, not every animal in Australia will hurt, kill or eat you. But be warned that some may, if they feel threatened or hungry, or if you prove Charles Darwin's natural selection theory correct because you got too close.

....

As athletes, we tend to be more active than most people; however, this doesn't mean we get outside or enjoy nature as much as we can or should.

....

A lot of our work and home lives may be indoors, which can lead to spending very little time enjoying the great outdoors. Humans have only been living predominantly inside and around concrete jungles for a couple of hundred years – if that – so maybe our brains still ache for nature because brain evolution doesn't work as fast as the town planners, architects and construction firms do.

Even when we do train and compete outside, it doesn't mean we notice our natural environment or take time to soak it in. It's often all around us, but our preoccupied brains can completely miss it. And that's unfortunate for your brain because nature is a positive and effective way for your active brain to recover and recharge.

FEELING GOOD IS ENOUGH REASON TO DO IT

There has been a lot of research into understanding why nature positively influences our brain's health, wellbeing and performance. While
we don't really understand why this is, the benefits are best summed
up by cognitive neuroscientist Dr David Strayer, who said that at 'the
end of the day, we come out in nature not because science says it does
something to us but because of how it makes us feel.' [54]

....

*We don't need to know why it feels good because that
doesn't change the positive experience we feel it has
on our brains.*

....

Unfortunately, many people spend most of the day and night with their
brains surrounded by walls, ceilings, air conditioning and various digital
screens. When we don't take a mental break outdoors, our brains miss
out on the chance to process our natural environments.

When we do get outside, we often rush from one place to the next
with no more than a cursory glance at our surroundings. As a result, we
miss out on these small but valuable opportunities to relax our brains
so that we feel mentally fresher for whatever is next on our busy plate.

As athletes, we love the positive chemical vibes from being physically
active, but we're not immune to missing out on nature's benefits even
when we're immersed in it all or most days. You miss out if your whole
time is spent focusing on smashing or surviving a session, hitting your
numbers, constantly monitoring your gadgets, talking non-stop with

your buddies (which has its own benefits), or trapped in your internal world as you pedal, push, run, roll, hit, jump or paddle your way from start to finish.

You might pause for a moment to take a selfie or a picture of the sunrise so you can post it with some funky caption, but how often do you pause for a few minutes and soak up nature just for yourself and in real-time?

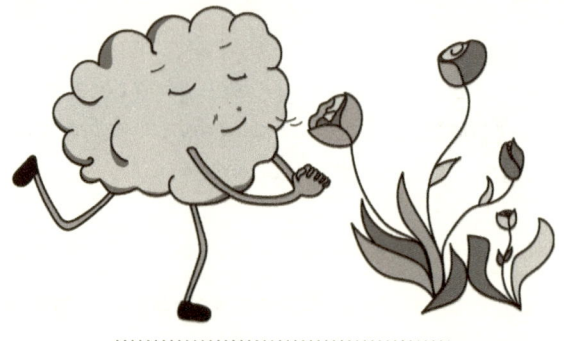

....

We miss out on opportunities to relax our brains and soak up what nature is offering us for free.

....

Nature can be found or created almost anywhere, but to be appreciated and provide a noticeable benefit, our brain needs to notice and dial into it. The phrase 'stop to smell the roses' is more than just a well-used metaphor for stopping to enjoy more of life's moments. In nature, when you don't stop and smell the roses or enjoy whatever else the great outdoors offers, it becomes another missed opportunity for your active brain to recover and recharge.

IT'S FREE ENERGY FOR YOUR BRAIN

Spending quality time in nature to help your brain recover and recharge doesn't have to cost a cent. A trade-off for our nature breaks is indeed time, but there are ways we can bring more activities to nature. For example, have a picnic instead of eating at a restaurant, or walk and talk with your friends instead of sitting in a pub or a coffee shop.

....

Aside from preferring to train and compete outdoors, I love spending other quality time outdoors.

....

I can feel my brain relaxing and thoughts becoming lighter within minutes of watching the trees in the wind, listening to the pouring rain, discovering shapes and objects in the clouds, sitting on the beach, or enjoying how birds sing and socialise. Spending time with nature helps boost my mood when I'm feeling flat, tired, frustrated, worried or sad.

Australian researchers analysed twenty-six peer-reviewed studies to better understand how different environments affect brain activity and mood. Studies 'reported that natural environments were positively experienced when compared to non-natural environments.' [55] These studies showed benefits experienced from spending time in green spaces, including:

- increased meditation, relaxation and engagement,
- recovery from brain fatigue,
- restoration of cognitive resources, and
- lower stress.

....

There is brain research that shows simply walking in nature may also help improve your mood, memory, attention and sleep.

....

A study led by Stanford University researchers in the US scanned the activity of participants' brains before and after a ninety-minute walk in either green or urban spaces. Participants who had their brain scanned after their walk through a green space 'showed increased activity in the subgenual prefrontal cortex, an area of the brain whose deactivation is affiliated with depression and anxiety – a finding that suggests nature may have important impacts on mood.'[54][56] This was not observed in the brains of people who walked through urban areas.

A recent review by researchers of studies spanning ten years found evidence of a connection between our exposure to nature and 'improved cognitive function, brain activity, blood pressure, mental health, physical activity, and sleep.'[57]

So, what do these findings mean for you and your brain? Not only can regular nature breaks help your brain recover and recharge to perform better as an athlete, but they also lift your mood and help you take more advantage of what your amazing brain can do for you in all areas of your life.

BOOST YOUR NEXT HARD EFFORT

There are times when a nature break for our brains must take a back seat to focusing on our performance if we want to do our best work and avoid an embarrassing or dangerous accident. Nonetheless, you can still soak up nature during a recovery session, while warming up or cooling down, while resting between hard efforts, and even during quiet moments in a race, game or event. These quick mental nature breaks can give your brain enough of a top up to help you shave off a couple of seconds, push out some extra watts, or go for a bit longer and further during your next focused effort.

....

Next time you rest your burning lungs and aching muscles between hard efforts, think about more than just letting your body recover. Give your brain some love too.

....

You already know the next set will be tough and will hurt, so instead of spending these moments worrying about that, which will also ramp up your brain's activity and stress levels, focus on taking in the sights, sounds and smells of nature around you.

TWO HOURS OF POWER IS QUALITY BRAIN TIME

You may wonder if there's evidence on how long and often you should take nature breaks for your brain to recover and recharge. You may already spend hours outside training, but how much of that do you need for your brain to benefit?

Let's check out a 2019 study of 20,000 participants to help answer this. Researchers concluded that after only 120 minutes in nature over a week, the participants reported their levels of health and wellbeing were 'significantly greater.' [58] These benefits still existed even when the two hours were broken into smaller chunks of time over a week.

....

Spending only two hours a week in nature is enough to help your brain. That's just over one per cent of your time in a week.

....

Researchers found no noticeable benefits when participants spent less than two hours a week in nature. And you don't need to spend half your waking hours in nature to have even greater results because no further benefits were observed above 300 minutes (five hours) a week. This gives us a guide that two to five hours spent in nature a week is enough to benefit your brain.

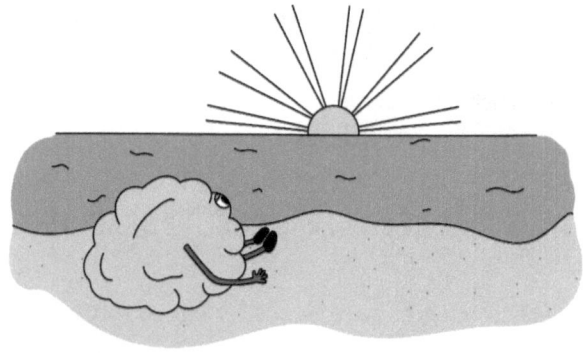

Two hours is just over one per cent of your time in a week, so complaining that you do not have enough time (in most cases) is a lame excuse. Another possible excuse is that nothing around you could be described as nature. While you may be spoiled for choice in Australia's Snowy Mountains, New Zealand's lakes or the French Pyrenees, nature breaks can be found in Melbourne, New York, Hong Kong, New Delhi, London, and anywhere else if you look.

If you look around your suburb or neighbourhood and discover parks, sports fields, rooftop gardens, front yards, grassed nature strips, trees, flowers, waterways or open spaces, you have found your opportunities for a nature break. It doesn't need to be spectacular scenery or a green oasis for your brain to benefit. We can always find some way to enjoy nature, but if you can't get outside for some reason, get some indoor plants to spruce things up and give your brain some green time.

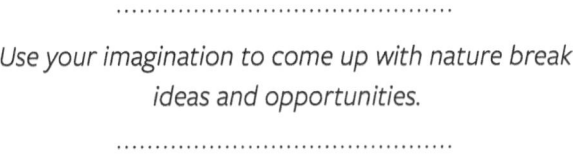

Use your imagination to come up with nature break ideas and opportunities.

There are no rules here. It can be as simple as taking short breaks from your office, home or anywhere else. If you find yourself indoors for long periods of time, go for a ten-minute wander outside. Don't take your phone, music, a book, work or other distractions with you. Just enjoy the trees, grass, sky, air, water and whatever else nature has gifted you in that place. Soak up what's around you.

Transitioning between your workplace and a training session can be a great opportunity to enjoy a few minutes of your natural surroundings so your brain has some downtime before you hit the track, pool, field, trails or court. This could be as simple as leaving your phone in your pocket while walking from your workplace to your car, bus, ferry, train or electric scooter.

By following these simple steps, you will make it as easy as possible for your brain to have nature breaks.

1. Write down a list of any outdoor activities you do now or could start doing. List whatever pops into your head – you aren't committing to any new activities yet.

2. Write a list of the natural and green spaces within a short distance of your home, workplace, university or wherever else you spend your days. Don't choose places that require you to drive in heavy traffic for miles or catch three train connections just to get there; this will make it unworkable to get your daily dose of nature.

3. Now choose an activity from step one that can be done at a location from step two. Choose a combination you can realistically and consistently achieve.

4. Using the following sentence example as your guide, write down how your new nature break will succeed. For example:

   'Every workday straight after I eat my lunch (when) **I** (who) **will go for a fifteen-minute walk without my phone** (what) **around the local park** (where).'

5. Return to step three until you plan to spend at least two hours of quality time experiencing nature every week.

CHAPTER HIGHLIGHTS

1. As athletes, we tend to be more active than most people; however, this doesn't mean we get outside or enjoy nature as much as we can or should.
2. Nature and green spaces can be found or created almost anywhere, but to be appreciated and provide a noticeable benefit, our brain needs to notice and dial into it.
3. While we may not understand precisely why nature feels good for us, just knowing this is enough to affect you and your brain positively.
4. Nature breaks can be experienced for free, and you only need to invest two to five hours weekly to benefit.
5. You can always find some way to enjoy nature, but if you can't get outside, get some indoor plants to spruce things up and give your brain some green time.

Chapter 9

Streamline Your Screentime

Prioritise recharging your brain over your smartphone

As a working athlete, I meet many other athletes and professionals who help keep us in shape so we can train, compete and move as freely and pain-free as possible. They include our coaches, physiotherapists, exercise physiologists and masseurs, who are often working athletes themselves.

I regularly get a sports massage, and there are generally sore spots, but I don't expect it to be as soothing as a half-day relaxation package at my local day spa. I find it a great opportunity to close my eyes, park my brain in a quieter place, and relax for the session. It's a great recovery opportunity for my tired brain, tender muscles and aching joints. I'll have a bit of chat but enjoy the silence too. The discomfort of the masseur's strong fingers and hard elbows makes me squirm sometimes, but I experience mostly good soreness.

I have a friend who is a sports masseur, and their job includes massaging players from professional sports teams. The players are full-time athletes and get a massage to help them recover from the physical toll that playing sport at the highest level takes on their bodies. I was talking about some brain-sciency stuff with my masseur friend and discovered that many of their athlete clients didn't switch off when they lie on the massage table. Instead, my friend said they spend most of their time on their smartphones playing games or consuming social media. These athletes are taking care of their body's recovery, but their brain is missing out. Rather than taking this perfect opportunity to wind down from a mentally and physically taxing job, their brain is working harder than they even realise.

DIGITAL SCREENS ARE EVERYWHERE

Like many athletes, our phones enable us to connect with other athletes and sporting communities worldwide. There are many positives that come from sharing our successes, disappointments and common interests with other athletes and supporters, so I'm not here to lecture or criticise our use of social media and other digital screen content.

....

Using social media enables us to connect with sporting communities almost anywhere around the world.

....

This chapter looks at the problem when we jump from one screen to another and don't take regular breaks. When your screentime habits exhaust your brain, your ability to be mentally switched on at training or in competition will be less than optimal, so your physical performance will suffer, regardless of how skilled, fit, tough, fast or strong you are. Cognitive neuroscientist Dr David Strayer, who studies how technology distracts our brains, explains, 'When you use your cell phone to talk, text, shoot photos, or whatever else you can do with your cell phone, you're tapping the prefrontal cortex and causing reductions in cognitive resources.' [54]

The prefrontal cortex (PFC) is in the forehead section of your brain and one of the most researched areas. Your PFC's performance is critical to your success as an athlete because it affects your working memory, which holds the information you consciously think about to plan and make decisions, predictions and judgements. It also helps us pay attention, assess risks and focus.

What Dr Strayer means is that using your phone and other screen gadgets drains your brain's energy quicker than you may realise, which means you have less energy available when you need it, like in a race or game where things aren't going as planned and you need to make smart adjustments to your strategy.

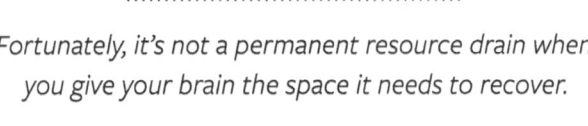

Fortunately, it's not a permanent resource drain when you give your brain the space it needs to recover.

When we 'go on a walk, without all of the gadgets, you've let the pre-frontal cortex recover,' continues Dr Strayer, 'and that's when we see these bursts in creativity, problem-solving, and feelings of wellbeing.' Leaving those screens behind can give your brain valuable opportunities to recover and perform.

A typical example of moving straight from one screen to another without a break is someone working at a computer who ducks away for fifteen minutes to grab a brew from their local coffee shop. Instead of giving their brain a break from the big screen they've been on for a couple of hours, they reach for their smartphone and use it while walking and talking, waiting to order, while they drink their brew, and on their way back to the office where another screen is waiting for their brain to return.

They've missed another opportunity that enables their brain to recover and recharge. Even if it's for just ten or fifteen minutes, staying away from screens positively affects how your brain feels. These smaller moments add up to make big changes in how you manage your brain's fatigue and energy.

WHY SCREENS DRAIN YOUR BRAIN'S ENERGY

Digital screens are where many of us do our work, have meetings, read, research, learn, watch videos, play games, shop, message each other, stay in contact with distant friends and family, chat with medical specialists, and entertain our brains. It's unrealistic, practically impossible and unwise to eliminate screens from our lives.

However, screen time without regular breaks creates brain fatigue problems because your brain is processing, interpreting and acting on the constant flow of information appearing on a screen. Often, we're working with new information or making new decisions about what to do with what's on our screen. In chapter one, we learned from Dr Barrett that these new experiences require your brain to work harder and use more fuel.

....

When you look at a screen, your eyes must continually refocus on a lot of small pixels ... just like the muscles that move your eyes get tired from all this work, so does your brain.

....

Another screentime fatigue factor is the increased workload on your eyes. When you look at a screen, your eyes must continually refocus on many small pixels that form the images and text, constantly changing as you scroll, flick, swipe, click, tap, pinch and speak at a screen. When your focus point is constantly changing like this, your brain works harder to make sense of the content. The muscles that move your eyes get tired from all this work, and so does your brain.

Your brain also gets bombarded by those annoying ads that appear after being sent by a cunning robot or algorithm tracking your online activity. You must decide what to do with those ads, which increases the demands on your brain.

All this refocusing by your eyes is collecting a tonne of data that your brain must process to make sense for you, which is the same for all your senses that interact with a digital screen. Making sense of everything your brain sees on a screen requires energy. The more complex the information and tired your brain is, the harder it is for your brain.

Eye specialist Dr Vicente Diaz from Yale School of Medicine agrees that it's more challenging work for your eyes to analyse and read screens than printed paper due to:

- reduced contrast between digital text and background,
- screen glare or reflection, and
- slightly blurry text on a screen. [59]

....

When you focus on a digital screen full of constantly changing pixels your eyes are working harder, and that means your neurons are doing more processing too.

....

DESIGNED TO GRAB YOUR BRAIN'S ATTENTION

A smartphone is generally our most used and accessible digital screen device. We use countless apps for social media, texting, emails, messaging, taking videos and photos, sharing posts and stories, surfing the web, doing work, analysing training stats, watching videos, and occasionally talking to people.

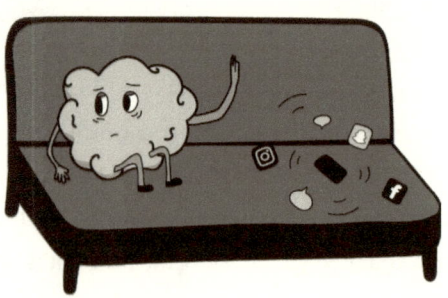

....

When something in your environment changes, your brain will notice whether you realise it or not ... the most effective trick is your phone's notifications.

....

Your smartphone and its apps attract your brain's attention with bright flashing colours, moving images, catchy sounds and vibrations. When something in your environment changes, your brain will notice – whether you realise it or not.

One of the most effective tricks that pulls your brain away from what it's paying attention to is your phone's notifications. Bright flashes, beeps and vibrations let your brain know there's something new on your phone. The phone grab and check are wired habits inside our brains.

The people who create content and screen gadgets are tapping into brain science to grab your attention, even if they don't understand how or realise they're doing it.

When your brain gets hooked on screen time by the cascading chemical and electrical signals bursting inside your head, you can feel like you've travelled twenty minutes into the future without realising it. It's easy to fall into the trap of spending more time on a screen than we planned, and we don't snap out of this trance until we're interrupted, our eyes and brain feel tired, we fall asleep, or we walk head first into a wall or light pole.

I still sometimes catch myself picking up my phone or jumping on my computer to check something and lose my awareness of time quickly. It's like my brain is hypnotised by the screen's content. And in a way it is, because the content was created to grab my brain's attention and to keep it there long enough to influence me to share posts, buy stuff, read blogs, listen to videos, follow people, or laugh at a meme that I'll probably steal and share if it matches my sense of humour.

People from all walks of life share content designed to steal your brain's attention, even if only for a few seconds. Driving while texting is just one example of when our brains' priorities become really messed up. Screen devices use various tricks to grab and hold your brain's attention against all the external competition, including whatever's going on in your head, even if it could kill you or someone else.

A chemical called dopamine gives us a feeling of pleasure when released into our brains, which can be triggered by our screens when we see some new activewear, order new running shoes, make it to the next level on our favourite online game, or see our finish line photo proudly posted on a social media page. These positive experiences encourage your brain to stay engaged with the screen longer to experience more pleasure, and to return more often to get another dose of dopamine.

....

When your brain associates pleasure with using your smartphone, it becomes a priority for your brain.

....

When you go to your phone more often and for longer to satisfy your brain's hunger, it becomes a top priority for your brain. If left unchecked, this cycle can drain your brain's energy – and your bank account if online shopping has you hooked.

Another chemical, called oxytocin, is often released when you experience a positive connection with another person or group. As working athletes, we tend to be connected to a team, club and community of like-minded athletes, officials and supporters. You may also follow your favourite professional athletes or team on social media and feel like you know them, even if you've never met them.

Your personal connections are important because they create good vibes that come from being accepted by others and belonging to a group, which has been integral to our ongoing survival as a species. Wanting to feel these experiences of acceptance and belonging is a reason we can spend more time online.

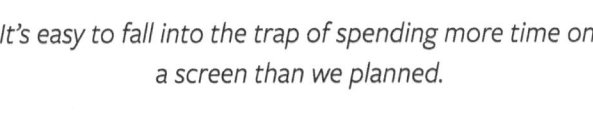

It's easy to fall into the trap of spending more time on a screen than we planned.

Stressful screentime experiences can trigger the release of chemicals, including adrenaline and cortisol, making us feel motivated, nervous, angry, focused or terrified. What we personally experience depends on how our brain processes and interprets the content, which will be different for you, me and everyone else. Our emotions and thoughts may be similar or at opposite ends of the spectrum. For example, watching a video of a mass swim start in a triathlon could nervously excite you, but terrify your squad mate.

Chemicals released in your brain and body can also give people a case of FOMO, or fear of missing out, a common threat that pulls them back to their screens repeatedly. A whole chapter in this book is about FOMO because it is a serious problem in becoming a Brainy Athlete.

The main point here is not the chemistry lesson on neurotransmitters and hormones released between your neurons or in your bloodstream.

The takeaway is that regardless of what chemicals are involved or why, it can lead to the same outcome: more screen time and an increased risk of becoming brain fatigued.

LIVING SMARTER WITH THEM, NOT WITHOUT

Screentime is here to stay because digital devices are a big part of our infrastructure and will only keep growing with technology. At least until we have a device planted in our heads and the data our brains process into images and words won't even need to be captured by our eyes first. Scary thought, but crazier science fiction has become a reality.

....

Our screens are a gateway to interacting with the real world in many useful ways.

....

There are many examples where technology has added value and allowed us to do so much more from almost anywhere in the world.

We can stay in touch and instantly share our lives, meet new lovers on dating apps, reach larger audiences to grow our businesses, access more opportunities to study almost anything, learn ways to become better athletes and watch live feeds of nearly every sport. We can know almost instantly when good and bad stuff happens worldwide, and anyone can become an online influencer who gets free stuff for looking cool and promoting it.

My approach to streamlining our screen time is to create good routines and habits that take back some of the lost time we spend on our screens. This includes having regular breaks that allow our brains to recover and recharge.

....

Changes to some of my routines have helped me make better decisions and create habits that streamline my screen time.

....

I usually don't need my smartphone attached to my hip, within arm's reach, or even in sight. When it is, I'm more likely to go for the automatic phone grab that can happen in the blink of an eye and before I can consciously stop it. I've found the out-of-reach or sight strategy effective for reducing my screen time because my brain must make a fresh decision about whether moving my body to open my bag or walk the ten steps to grab my phone is worth the energy needed.

This strategy works for me while I'm at my desk, in bed, on the couch, in a café chatting with friends, waiting in line at a shop, walking the streets, as a passenger in a car, bus or train, and even going to the toilet. The toilet is where many people add to their screen time, not that I've been actively researching or recording my experiences in public restrooms. I'll rely on a couple of surveys instead.

A 2021 American survey published by Vioguard found seventy-three per cent of 1,100 people 'admitted to using their phone on the toilet or standing at the urinal, regardless of age or gender.'[60] A study of 500 Australians also found that forty per cent use their phone in the bathroom.[61] If brain fatigue isn't scary enough to stop you from disconnecting from your phone while on the toilet, think about the hygiene risks you're taking with you once you leave the bathroom.

....

I've learned to be more comfortable separating myself from my phone when I don't need it and it's safe to do so.

....

When I take our dog for a walk around the block, I almost always leave my phone at home. That way, I'm removing the temptation of that automatic phone grab. Instead, my brain loves sharing our dog's adventures and soaking up nature, which is a strategy discussed in another chapter. If there is an emergency while walking our dog, I don't need my phone for help. I can simply knock on someone's door, yell for help, or throw dog poo at someone if they're chasing me.

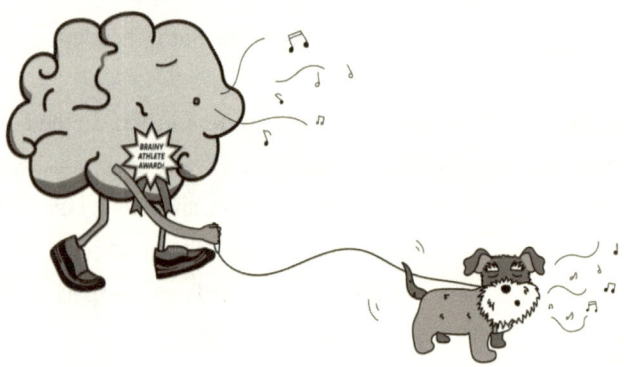

I've turned off all the notifications on my phone except for calls, texts and calendar reminders. I became fed up with the constant beeping and vibrating long ago. I've blocked most phone notifications appearing on my watch and bike computer because if my watch or bike pings, it's a distraction from my training that could also end in an embarrassing or nasty accident. There may be reasons you need your phone to announce certain notifications, but think about reducing how many are turned on.

....

Having regular breaks during your workday to break free from your constant screentime can be achieved if you schedule it as a priority and set yourself little reminders to do it.

....

You can use a stopwatch, download apps or software that remind you to give your brain a break, or create music playlists that go for around forty-five minutes. When the playlist stops, so do you. Use your imagination to come up with interesting or fun ways to remind you to take a break, or get out the old-school egg timer if that works for you.

If you have control over other people's time and energy, you have an added responsibility to consider more than just your brain. I have learned over time how important it is to include regular breaks and mix up the delivery style in workshops and coaching sessions.

A brain-fatigued client becomes bored and disengaged, and misses out on making the most of their opportunity to learn and develop. I usually throw in a five-minute break every forty-five minutes, with much longer breaks mid-morning, at lunch, and mid-afternoon.

If you run online or face-to-face training, meetings, webinars, or anything similar, include some breaks for everyone's brain to gear down and recover. Smash them with too much for too long, and everyone, including you, suffers.

There are loads of other options that can help you reduce your screen-time so your brain can recover and recharge. Check them out online, but don't stay there too long without a break. Find what you're looking for, watch a cute animal video, and then do something that doesn't require screen time. Your eyes and brain will thank you for it.

CHAPTER HIGHLIGHTS

1. Digital screens are here to stay and are a gateway to interacting with the world in many valuable ways.

2. When you jump from one screen to another without regular breaks, your brain will struggle to help you perform at your athletic best.

3. Your eye focus constantly changes when looking at a digital screen. This tires your eyes and your brain.

4. Create good habits that look after your brain by taking back some of the lost time spent on your screens to have regular breaks. Simply walking without your phone and other gadgets helps your brain recover.

5. Don't use your phone on the toilet. It'll drain your brain and contaminate your phone. Read the messages on the back of the toilet door instead.

Chapter 10

Be Less Mind-full

Controlling your attention is a superpower

One of the most impressive winter sports for me is the biathlon, which combines cross-country skiing with rifle shooting. Biathletes skate a few laps around a set course with their rifle slung over their shoulder, and on each lap they stop and shoot at targets fifty metres away. If they miss a shot, they receive a time penalty. The winner is the athlete with the lowest overall time, so skiing fast and shooting accurately is a good strategy.

One reason I'm impressed by biathletes is that although I've never skied cross-country, I am a downhill skier, and it can be hard work just skating twenty metres across the snow to get on a lift. Biathletes need to skate for up to twenty kilometres in a race, on undulating terrain, without constant help from gravity, and it's usually freezing.

Another reason I'm impressed is their ability to shoot accurately immediately after completing each lung-burning and energy-sapping lap. Just imagine their racing heartbeat, heaving chest and burning legs as they look over their rifle at a tiny target fifty metres away. The clock is ticking, and a miss will add more time; competitors are moving around you, and it still feels like Siberia in mid-winter. No pressure at all. Somehow, they calm themselves down enough to provide a stable and focused platform to shoot and hit the targets. Most of the time, anyway.

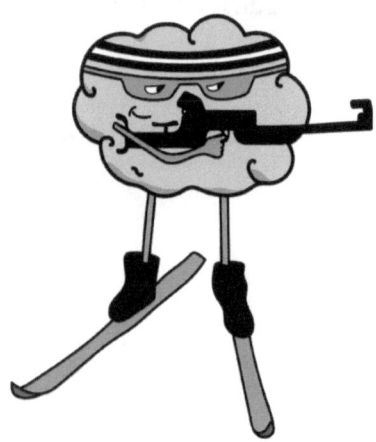

I have so much respect for biathletes because I've trained with rifles in the police, and it's not easy to remain calm and focused when the pressure's on during a qualification assessment or high-stress scenario. If you can't relax when you're breathing heavily and your heart rate's increasing, it's easy to miss and fail a test, which isn't helpful for your job or confidence. If Olympic biathletes miss a shot because their breathing is uncontrolled or they lose focus, that can mean the difference between a gold medal and a bronze or silver, or receiving no award at all.

....

Not only must biathletes manage their body's response to physical exertion, they must also calm their mind.

....

Precision is essential to shoot successfully, and a biathlete's attention must be focused on hitting the next target. They can use their mind to relax their body and vice versa. If they start thinking about the shot they just missed, how many laps are left, who is next to them, or what's for dinner, there's a good chance they'll miss. It is true that many athletes train frequently and replicate their technical skills repeatedly, so they perform well under pressure. However, they are also human, and when doubt or distraction creeps into their thoughts, even the most skilled and experienced athletes can stumble.

I was a firearms instructor in the police, and if an officer's attention was focused on not missing the target instead of hitting it, they would often miss. And if they worried more about failing an assessment instead of concentrating on the effectiveness of each shot, they often failed. What we pay attention to and focus on often becomes our reality. Therefore, a pathway to success for biathletes, police and anyone else is to pay more attention to what's helpful and what you want instead of what's unhelpful and what you don't want. Unhelpful thoughts and behaviours are distractions to performing at our athletic best and can come from anywhere in our life and at any time.

YOU HAVE BEEN PAYING ATTENTION, BUT WHERE?

Mindfulness, to me, is simply attention control – the skill of being aware of your thoughts, choosing where they go, and moving them to where you need them to be. As you become more present, rather than drifting to the past and future, you become more in tune with your internal and external environment and more aware of what you're experiencing now, which is where you can make the most difference.

While meditation and mindfulness are closely linked, they are not the same. Ariel Garten is a co-founder of the company Muse, which manufactures innovative products we can use at home to help us meditate. Garten explains, 'Meditation is a practice, or training, that leads to healthy and positive mindsets. Mindfulness is a skill that is built as a result.' He says, 'Meditation builds the skill of mindfulness.' [62.] I agree with this differentiation between mindfulness and meditation.

The connection between meditation and mindfulness is comparable to the relationship between your training and competition. They're different, but you can't expect to execute your skills and compete physically if you don't practice at training. Likewise, you can't expect to effectively control your attention when necessary if you don't train through meditation.

....

Learning to control your attention can become your superpower, just like it has for many other athletes, including me.

....

Attention control is a superpower that intersects every part of our lives, including business, sports, relationships, learning and leadership. It's a superpower because it helps you direct your brain's precious energy towards what is most helpful at that point in time. By guiding your attention, you're likely to waste less energy and time on what is unhelpful and irrelevant to supporting your athletic performance.

....

Attention control is one of the foundational skills I mentor and coach athletes and leaders to develop.

....

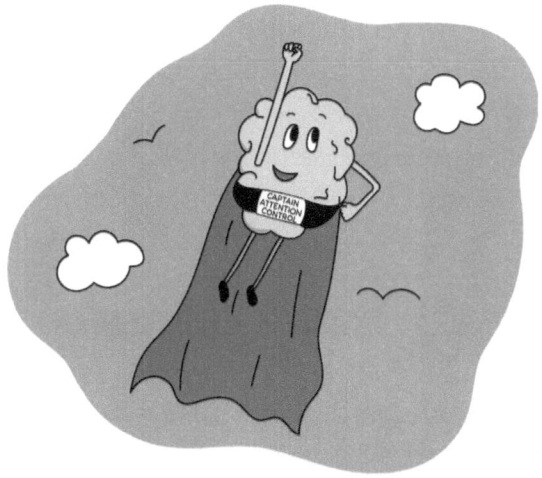

Attention control creates a clearer and sharper mind, and this was a skill I worked with Aussie cricketer Maitlan Brown to develop. She describes her experience like this, 'I'm noticing a clearer mindset around training and a deeper understanding of my development as both a player and a person.' Improving her attention control has given Maitlan a superpower that transcends her cricket and affects all areas of her life.

Attention control can be applied to any sector of your life, including your sport. For example, I learned to practise meditation at home, but the attention skills I have developed can be applied anytime. As these skills have developed, so have my empathy, active listening, emotional regulation, confidence, calmness, focus, sense of humour and awareness.

My tendency to ruminate about the past, worry excessively about the future, and indulge other distractions, has diminished. I also notice my thoughts and feelings much earlier than I used to because I'm less distracted. When those thoughts and feelings are unhelpful, noticing them earlier means I can acknowledge them and move on a lot easier and sooner, and before my negative thoughts get out of control. I used to have a very active brain, but now I am more relaxed, which means my brain has more opportunities to relax and recover, so I have more cognitive resources and energy available when I really need them.

BETTER CHOICES FOR YOUR PRECIOUS TIME AND ENERGY

Attention control is a superpower for better choices about using your time and brain's energy. It helps you allocate these two limited and precious resources to the highest priorities that exist in the present moment. That could be resting, setting your bike up in transition, chatting to a friend, planning your race, warming up in the nets, practising a new skill, or studying the competition. Wherever you are right now, that's where you have the biggest influence and can make the biggest difference. What you think and do directly impacts what happens next and how well you perform as an athlete today and tomorrow.

Headspace creates science-backed meditation and mindfulness tools to help develop your attention control. In an online article, sports psychologist Dr Kristin Keim says, 'A mind that is not under control is a mind that makes mistakes – mistakes that could prevent you from winning.' [63] One of the key techniques she draws on to help athletes is meditation. Dr Keim explains that the benefits athletes can reap from meditation include:

- stress reduction – your body will learn how to relax in stressful situations,
- improved sleep patterns and quicker recovery time,

- enhanced endurance – you can train yourself to go harder and for longer, and
- improvement in your mind-body connection, helping you to discover your optimal performance zone.

Sleep is essential for your survival and for your brain's recovery and performance. It's not uncommon for athletes to feel restless or anxious the night before a race or game. The physiological changes we experience can be interpreted by our brain in various ways. For example, you could interpret these changes as positive experiences, such as excitement, or you can dread them as a feeling of fear. Either way, your thoughts are making that choice, and attention control is a superpower to help quieten your active brain and body so you can sleep.

Imagine if you had the superpower of mindfulness to either consolidate your positive thoughts or move away from negativity. This can change the chemistry in your body, but even if it didn't, you could at least think more positively about what you're feeling. Anxiousness can become excitement. Concern can become a methodical pre-race plan. You experience more choices when you can control your attention.

....

You fight less against the chemistry inside and turn your attention to what thoughts and behaviours are helpful.

....

Let's look at the example of the biathlete. They can use mindfulness to transition successfully from a missed shot to thinking only about the next shot they need to take. You can also use this technique to your advantage if you're a runner, triathlete, cricketer, footballer, swimmer, rower or any other athlete. It's a superpower that will help you before, during, and after training and competition because you can make better decisions at each moment.

Many of us spend a lot of time and brain energy on our phones and computers without giving our brains enough breaks to rest and recover. If screentime has become an automatic behaviour for you, you may not know how deeply it affects you. When you're focused on your device's content, it's easy for time to fly by and your brain to feel fatigued.

Our screen devices are the platform for what is probably our greatest distraction today. Improving your attention control through meditation and mindfulness is a valuable skill that will help you perform and choose where to spend your brain's energy.

MY FAST TRACK TO GREATER ATTENTION CONTROL

I've lost count of how many times I've been asked over the years, 'Are you listening?' or 'Have you been paying attention to anything I've said?' I often wasn't because I was easily distracted, caught up in my thoughts, and rarely present. I still get asked these questions, but less often because the practice of meditation and the skill of mindfulness have become top priorities for me over the past three years.

....

I call attention control a superpower in this chapter because that's precisely what I believe it is.

....

But I haven't always thought this way. In fact, it's only been the last three years that it's become a vital part of my life. And lucky for me, from the outset, I was introduced to remarkable technology that we can use anywhere to learn meditation and improve our mindfulness or attention control skills.

In 2019, I was in Melbourne as a student completing the i4 Neuroleader Certification that was created by the About my Brain Institute. Silvia and Relmi Damiano are the creative and passionate brains behind it, and this certification was the starting point in my journey into the human brain. I am grateful to Silvia and Relmi for their support, friendship and shared passion for the brain.

I had the opportunity to wear a personal neurofeedback device during this program to measure my brain activity while practising meditation. I had never heard of these devices and knew little about brain activity, but I was curious to try it. Neurofeedback technology allows us to scan our brain waves, or the electrical activity in our brain, in real time. We can use the feedback to practise meditation. This then improves our mindfulness skills. It's brain training for attention control.

I was excited and astonished by the experience at the program, and a couple of months later I purchased my own home neurofeedback device. I describe it as a plastic headband with sensors on the inside that can read my brainwave activity from the surface of my head. To practise meditation, I turn it on, put it on my forehead and over my ears, and connect it via Bluetooth to the app on my phone. I choose what soundscape or guided meditation option I want to listen to and how long my session is. Once it calibrates its sensors to my brain waves, I start meditating. At the end of the session, it provides a readout in the app of what my brain activity was. It's just like reading the fitness data on your smartwatch at the end of a training session.

I only occasionally use the device because I have a strong practical understanding of meditating without it. I show it at many of my workshops and presentations and have lent it to some clients for trial. One of my professional athlete clients recently borrowed it for a few days. As a result, they ordered their own device.

....

My attention control wouldn't be close to where it is today without learning with a neurofeedback device.

....

There are plenty of phone apps and other resources that can help you practice meditation and develop your mindfulness skills, and these can be effective too. Apps like these may be all you need. My experience with personal neurofeedback technology resulted in my practice being more consistent, and I was able to measure and track my development and grow my skills quicker and more effectively.

Whatever your approach to practising meditation and developing your mindfulness skill, you can make attention control your superpower and reap the benefits of becoming a Brainy Athlete.

CAN WE MULTITASK?

You can complete multiple automatic behaviours simultaneously because your brain's neural networks for those actions have been strongly developed through your practice and repetition. Examples of athletes' automated actions include many of the technical skills they have worked on for years, but this isn't unique. Learning a habit is how our brains conserve energy and free up the limited resources available for conscious thought.

However, when you're doing a complex or new task that isn't automatic, your brain can't multitask in the way you may think. 'When we talk about multitasking, we are really talking about attention: the art of paying attention, the ability to shift our attention, and, more broadly, to exercise judgement about what objects are worthy of our attention,' says Dr Gillian Clark of the cognitive neuroscience unit, Deakin University, Australia. [64]

Dr Clark says, 'One way our brain can deal with this problem is by switching between tasks. This can feel as though we're focusing on multiple things at once, but our brain is more likely focusing on one thing, switching to another, switching back, and so on.'

I'm not saying there aren't people whose brains can process information in ways that can't be explained and could be doing something like multitasking. For example, neurodiversity, or variations in how individual brains function, shows that some brains can do remarkable things we don't fully understand and in ways that most of us can't.

For most of us, paying attention to one non-automatic task at a time will save time and energy and put us in the best position to absorb the information accurately and thoroughly.

CHAPTER HIGHLIGHTS

1. Meditation trains you in the skill of mindfulness or attention control.

2. Attention control is a superpower that gives you more significant influence over your thoughts, feelings and actions.

3. Being more in tune with your attention helps you identify and influence where your energy is on the BEC.

4. Technology can help you fast track your skill development.

5. Attention control helps athletes rest and recover when not training or competing, and helps them perform when they are.

Conclusion:

Your Brainy Athlete Investment

'As athletes, we often prioritise our physical, technical and tactical needs but never really take time to work on the most important thing... our brain!' This was shared by English cricketer Tammy Beaumont following her decision to become one of my many inspirational clients and someone I now call a friend. Tammy has an exceptional athletic career that includes being 2019 Wisden Cricketer of the Year, 2017 Women's Cricket World Cup Player of the Tournament, 2021 ICC Women's T20 Cricketer of the Year, and a National Schools Gymnastics Champion.

As we continue to work together, Tammy has experienced positive shifts in her relationship with her brain because she has taken steps to prioritise it both on and off the cricket field.

Tammy's experience strengthened my confidence to put me on the right track for this book. When I decided to write this book, my main goal was to enrich your relationship with your brain. It's the only one you'll ever have, and your athletic performance and health are highly dependent on the strength of your relationship with your brain and your priority on taking care of it.

I didn't understand much about my brain or what it needed from me until I threw myself headfirst, or maybe brain first, into learning as much as I could about it. Before then, I rarely thought about my brain, and I certainly didn't feel affection for it. It was out of sight, out of mind, and I didn't treat it as a priority. I took my brain for granted without realising how much I was missing out on and how I was neglecting it.

I had to write this book because I figured that most people, including you, probably have a more distant relationship with their brains than they should. Because of what I've experienced for several years and the significant benefits to my clients and me, I wanted to share my understanding with you and anyone else who wants to become a Brainy Athlete.

I wanted to do much more than write a book about a bunch of strategies and include tips to help change some of your behaviours. While our behaviours deliver change, they often become automatic or routine, which means you don't pay much attention to them. While you will benefit from better habits and routines and your brain having to use less energy to drive them, expanding your awareness and continual development comes with a fundamental shift in how you think about your brain.

At the start of this book, I challenged you to change how you think about your brain and to build a more loving relationship with it. I wonder if you have, even just a little, and if it's a relationship you believe is valuable enough to prioritise and continue investing in. If you have, your brain will feel loved and continue to grow and do its best to support you, your athletic goals, and every other area of your life.

Eliud Kipchoge is a Kenyan Olympian athlete who in 2019 famously broke the two-hour barrier for a marathon by twenty seconds. This was a monumental achievement as he became the first human to run that distance under two hours. It didn't count as an official record because it didn't follow normal race conditions and, remarkably, Kipchoge's fastest official time in a marathon is the world record time and only sixty-nine seconds above two hours.

Kipchoge is not your average athlete, but he is still human and, just like us, his performance and wellbeing is influenced by the biological limitations of his brain and body. And based on what he has been quoted saying, he prioritises his brain and respects it as much, if not more, than the legs that have made him the fastest marathoner in history. The following are a selection of quotes by Kipchoge that demonstrate he is a Brainy Athlete who prioritises his brain.

- *'Athletics is not so much about the legs. It's about the heart and mind.'* [65]
- *'If you want to break through, your mind should be able to control your body. Your mind should be a part of your fitness.'* [66]
- *'In the offseason I allow my body to recover, my mind to recover. I like to be with my family, to read books, and know what is going on in the world, to understand how people think.'* [67]
- *My average sleeping hours is ten hours. I sleep for eight hours at night, and two during the day.'* [68]

Now that you've come to the end of this book and made a conscious and deliberate decision to be a Brainy Athlete, it's time to put what you've learned towards creating a strategy that inspires you to prioritise your brain.

The following ten questions capture the essence of the corresponding ten chapters in this book. They're designed to turn your thoughts into actions. As you answer each question, reflect on what you've read and learned, what you already knew, and what is possible. You don't have to have a plan yet to answer these questions. Let your brain run free to come up with answers to each question and then you can move onto creating a strategy. My website gazmills.com/brainyresources has extra resources to help you come up with your ideas and put them into action.

1. What can you do to influence your brain's energy flow to the right of the BEC?
2. What can you do to bring your brain into sight and mind more often?
3. What can you do to spice up your brain's experiences?
4. What can you do differently to keep your brain's eye on the prize?
5. What can you do to feel more alive and live your life, not someone else's?
6. What can you prioritise tonight, so you show up stronger tomorrow?
7. What fuel choices can you make to start and stay sharp?
8. Where can you take your brain for regular breaks with nature?
9. What can you do differently to prioritise your brain over your screen devices?
10. What can you do to make attention control your superpower?

Nobody will realise 100 per cent of their brain's potential for various reasons, but that doesn't mean you need to be at 100 per cent performance to succeed at your sport or in any other area of your life.

To continue your Brainy Athlete journey, just like Tammy, Maitlan and many of my other amazing clients, answer these ten questions right now. Perfection is not your goal, prioritising your brain to help you be the best athlete you can be is. Trust me; your brain will thank you for it!

Acknowledgments

Firstly, to my wife, Nicole, thank you for your encouragement, patience and love, and helping me strike a balance between spreading my wings and being grounded. It hasn't always been easy, but anything that's worth it generally isn't. To Angus and Elleri, your years may be young, but you have both taught me so much about what really matters in life. Thank you also to the rest of my family, who have all played a big role in who I am today.

To my publishing gurus from Grammar Factory Publishing who believed in me and helped bring my book to life. Thank you Scott, Olivia, Carolyn, Ania, Julia, Dania and the rest of the team who supported me.

To my book coach, Kelly Irving from the Expert Author Academy, thank you for being my expert guide and loving critic as I navigated my way from knowing nothing about writing a book to becoming a published author.

To Sophia Meldrum, thank you for your artistic genius at bringing the Brainy Athlete illustrations to life in this book and for your valuable feedback as a former elite athlete.

Thank you Maitlan, James, Dave, Tammy, Megan, Martin, Angela and Vikki for making time in your busy lives to read my book and write a testimonial. What you and your brains have achieved inspires me.

To everyone who has supported me and been a sounding board since I first floated the idea of writing a book nearly three years ago, a massive thank you. Your words of encouragement and interest in my author journey have been confidence boosters and motivators to keep me going and give my best to this book.

A special thank you to Lauren, Davey and Maitlan for your raw and honest feedback on the very early versions of my book and thought bombs. Thank you to Silvia and Relmi, and to Rob, for your friendship and mentoring in my journey to love and understand more about my brain.

Thank you, Erik Severson, for including me in my first opportunity to become a published author in our Amazon best-selling book, *Peak Performance: Mindset Tools for Business*.

To all my clients, customers and partners, thank you for your trust in our partnership.

And finally, to you, thank you for your decision to take this life-changing step to become a Brainy Athlete. Whatever your sport and the level you compete at, you and your fellow athletes push the boundaries to bridge the gap between possibility and reality.

About the author

Gaz Mills is a Neurocoach, speaker and author who simplifies brain science to develop brainy athletes, leaders and teams. He wants everyone to have a more loving and understanding relationship with their brain.

Gaz founded Garry Mills Peak Performance in 2016 and his philosophy is 'Leadership and wellbeing is not rocket science. It's brain science.' ®

He has facilitated, coached and presented for thousands of people in workshops, conferences, training programs and other events.

His clients include world-class professional and elite athletes, passionate leaders, entrepreneurs and teams across the private and public sectors. They have described his services as interactive, insightful, fun and light-hearted. Gaz blends neuroscience with everything he's learned and experienced to offer unique and real-world opportunities for personal and professional growth. With twenty-five years of diverse and extensive experience across the public and private sectors, including leading complex and sensitive operations in Australia and overseas, he has led large teams and achieved critical training and operational outcomes for large organisations. Previous experiences include being a bodyguard to the Australian Prime Minister, a specialist police officer and a training team manager.

His qualifications include the Fundamentals of Neuroscience Program awarded by Harvard online and a Professional Coach Program recognised by the International Coach Federation. He is also a co-author of an Amazon best-selling book, *Peak Performance: Mindset Tools for Business.*

Gaz has been an amateur athlete for most of his life, growing up playing cricket and footy in country New South Wales, Australia. In recent years he has trained and competed in rowing, long-distance triathlon, endurance running and road cycling. Gaz is married to another keen athlete, Nicole, and they live in Canberra and Broulee, Australia. He has two adult children, Angus and Elleri.

You can connect with Gaz or get in touch by visiting the following links.

- gazmills.com
- @gaz_mills
- linkedin.com/in/gaz-mills-39b18878
- gaz@gazmills.com

References and citations

A massive thank you to the scientists, researchers, authors, organisations, publishers and other experts whose incredible work has contributed to my book. I have done my best to attribute your research and publications to the correct source and I sincerely apologise if I've made a mistake or left someone out.

Chapter 1

1 Feldman Barrett, L., & Quigley, K. S. (2021, July 15). *Interoception: The secret ingredient*. Dana Foundation. Retrieved January 10, 2023, from https://www.dana.org/article/interoception-the-secret-ingredient/

2 Feldman Barrett, D. L. (2022, June 28). *How emotions trick your brain*. BBC Science Focus Magazine. Retrieved January 10, 2023, from https://www.sciencefocus.com/the-human-body/how-emotions-trick-your-brain-2/

3 Slimani, M., Znazen, H., Bragazzi, N. L., Zguira, M. S., & Tod, D. (2018, December 3). *The effect of mental fatigue on cognitive and aerobic performance in adolescent active endurance athletes: Insights from a randomized. counterbalanced, cross-over trial*. Journal of clinical medicine. Retrieved January 10, 2023, from https://www.ncbi.nlm.nih.gov/pmc/articles/PMC6306934/

4 Zhang D., Li J., Miller R., Batraka M., Effing S., Hossain F., Bernard A., Marillier M. and Domnik N. (2021). Are Your Muscles or Your Brain Making You Feel Tired After Exercise? Front. Young Minds. 9:578431. Retrieved January 10, 2023, from https://kids.frontiersin.org/articles/10.3389/frym.2021.578431#KC5a

5 Carroll T.J., Taylor J.L., Gandevia S.C. (2017, May 1). Recovery of central and peripheral neuromuscular fatigue after exercise. J Appl Physiol; Retrieved January 10, 2023, from https://journals.physiology.org/doi/pdf/10.1152/japplphysiol.00775.2016

6 American Physiological Society. (2009, February 26). *Mental fatigue can affect physical endurance*. ScienceDaily. Retrieved January 10, 2023, from https://www.sciencedaily.com/releases/2009/02/090224132915.htm

7 Feldman Barrett, L. (2021, March 4). *Variation is the stuff of life. So why can it make us uncomfortable?* The Guardian. Retrieved January 10, 2023, from https://www.theguardian.com/commentisfree/2021/mar/04/variation-uncomfortable-embracing-difference-success-species

8 The Hub Staff. (2022, February 14). *Neuroscientist Lisa Feldman Barrett demystifies the brain*. The Hub. Retrieved January 10, 2023, from https://thehub.ca/2022-02-14/neuroscientist-lisa-feldman-barrett-demystifies-the-brain/

9 Jabr, F. (2012, July 18). *Does thinking really hard burn more calories?* Scientific American. Retrieved January 10, 2023, from https://www.scientificamerican.com/article/thinking-hard-calories/

10 Olsen, K. (2020, March 17). *Your brain at work*. NeuroLeadership Institute. Retrieved January 10, 2023, from https://neuroleadershipinstitute.org/2020/03/17/while-we-all-work-from-home-cozy-up-to-cognitive-capacity/

Chapter 2

11 *Glutamate: What it is & function*. Cleveland Clinic. (n.d.). Retrieved January 10, 2023, from https://my.clevelandclinic.org/health/articles/22839-glutamate

12 Wiehler, A., Branzoli, F., Adanyeguh, I., Mochel, F., & Pessiglione, M. (2022, August 11). *A neuro-metabolic account of why daylong cognitive work alters the control of economic decisions*. Current Biology. Retrieved January 10, 2023, from https://www.sciencedirect.com/science/article/abs/pii/S0960982222011113

13 Saha, N., Cuffari, B. (2022, August 16). *Here's why thinking hard exhausts you*. News-Medical.net. Retrieved January 10, 2023, from https://www.news-medical.net/news/20220815/Heres-why-thinking-hard-exhausts-you.aspx

14 Heads up. (n.d.). *What is good mental health?* What is good mental health. Retrieved January 10, 2023, from https://www.headsup.org.au/your-mental-health/what-is-good-mental-health

Chapter 3

15 Pires, F. O., Silva-Júnior, F. L., Brietzke, C., Franco-Alvarenga, P. E., Pinheiro, F. A., de França, N. M., Teixeira, S., & Meireles Santos, T. (2018, March 1). *Mental fatigue alters cortical activation and psychological responses, impairing performance in a distance-based cycling trial*. Frontiers. Retrieved January 10, 2023, from https://www.frontiersin.org/articles/10.3389/fphys.2018.00227/full

Chapter 4

16 Lee, S., Charles, S. T., & Almeida, D. M. (2021, June 14). *Change is good for the brain: Activity diversity and cognitive functioning across adulthood*. The journals of gerontology. Series B, Psychological sciences and social sciences. Retrieved January 10, 2023, from https://www.ncbi.nlm.nih.gov/pmc/articles/PMC8200355/

17 Scarmeas, N., & Stern, Y. (2003, August). *Cognitive Reserve and lifestyle.* Journal of clinical and experimental neuropsychology. Retrieved January 10, 2023, from https://www.ncbi.nlm.nih.gov/pmc/articles/PMC3024591/

18 Stern, Y. (2002, March). *What is Cognitive Reserve? Theory and research application of the reserve concept.* Journal of the International Neuropsychological Society: JINS. Retrieved January 10, 2023, from https://pubmed.ncbi.nlm.nih.gov/11939702/

19 Fancourt, D., & Steptoe, A. (2019, February 28). *Television viewing and cognitive decline in older age: Findings from the English Longitudinal Study of Ageing.* Scientific reports. Retrieved January 10, 2023, from https://pubmed.ncbi.nlm.nih.gov/30820029/

20 Cowper, W. (1785). *The task, a poem to which are added an epistle to Joseph Hill, Tirocinium; or, a review of schools, and the history of John Gilpin.* Printed for J. Johnson.

Chapter 5

21 Clear, J. (2018). *Atomic Habits.* Random House Business Books.

22 Gustafson, C., & Lipton PhD, B. (2017, December). *Bruce Lipton, PhD: The jump from cell culture to consciousness.* Integrative medicine (Encinitas, Calif.). Retrieved January 10, 2023, from https://www.ncbi.nlm.nih.gov/pmc/articles/PMC6438088/

23 Thaler, R. H., & Sunstein, C. R. (2009). *Nudge: Improving decisions about health, wealth and happiness.* Penguin.

Chapter 6

24 Andrew K. Przybylski, Kou Murayama, Cody R. DeHaan, Valerie Gladwell, (2013, April 9). *Motivational, emotional, and behavioral correlates of fear of missing out.* Computers in Human Behavior. Retrieved January 10, 2023, from https://www.sciencedirect.com/science/article/abs/pii/S0747563213000800?via%3Dihub

25 Grohol, J. (2022, March 31). *FOMO: Causes and solutions.* Psych Central. Retrieved January 10, 2023, from https://psychcentral.com/health/what-is-fomo-the-fear-of-missing-out#effects

26 Laurence, E., & Temple, J. (2022, September 30). *The psychology behind the fear of missing out (FOMO).* Forbes. Retrieved January 10, 2023, from https://www.forbes.com/health/mind/the-psychology-behind-fomo/

Chapter 7

27 SHF Australia. (2021, August 12). *Asleep on the job: Costs of inadequate sleep in

Australia. The Sleep Health Foundation. Retrieved January 10, 2023, from https://www.sleephealthfoundation.org.au/news/special-reports/asleep-on-the-job-costs-of-inadequate-sleep-in-australia.html

28 Commonwealth of Australia. (2019, April). *Bedtime reading - sleep.org.au*. Retrieved January 10, 2023, from https://www.sleep.org.au/common/Uploaded%20 files/Public%20Files/About/BedtimeReading.pdf

29 SHF Australia. (2016, August 5). *How much sleep do you really need?* The Sleep Health Foundation. Retrieved January 10, 2023, from https://www.sleephealthfoundation.org.au/how-much-sleep-do-you-really-need.html

30 Paprocki, J. (2009, August 14). *The "Short sleep" gene: When six hours is enough.* American Academy of Sleep Medicine, Sleep Education. Retrieved January 10, 2023, from https://sleepeducation.org/short-sleep-gene-when-six-hours-enough/

31 Chai, Y., Fang, Z., Yang, F. N., Xu, S., Deng, Y., Raine, A., Wang, J., Yu, M., Basner, M., Goel, N., Kim, J. J., Wolk, D. A., Detre, J. A., Dinges, D. F., & Rao, H. (2020, May 29). *Two nights of recovery sleep restores hippocampal connectivity but not episodic memory after total sleep deprivation*. Nature News. Retrieved January 11, 2023, from https://www.nature.com/articles/s41598-020-65086-x

32 Suni, E., & Vyas, N. (2022, December 16). *How lack of sleep impacts cognitive performance and focus.* Sleep Foundation. Retrieved January 11, 2023, from https://www.sleepfoundation.org/sleep-deprivation/lack-of-sleep-and-cognitive-impairment

33 Skiba, V., & Matsumura, A. (2020, December). *Insufficient sleep syndrome.* American Academy of Sleep Medicine, Sleep Education. Retrieved January 11, 2023, from https://sleepeducation.org/sleep-disorders/insufficient-sleep-syndrome/

34 Tornero-Aguilera, J. F., Jimenez-Morcillo, J., Rubio-Zarapuz, A., & Clemente-Suárez, V. J. (2022, March 25). *Central and peripheral fatigue in physical exercise explained: A narrative review*. International journal of environmental research and public health. Retrieved January 12, 2023, from https://www.ncbi.nlm.nih.gov/pmc/articles/PMC8997532/

35 Lock A.M., Bonetti D.L., & Campbell A.D.K. (2018, November). *The psychological and physiological health effects of fatigue.* Occupational medicine (Oxford, England). Retrieved January 12, 2023, from https://pubmed.ncbi.nlm.nih.gov/30445654/

36 Whitney, P., Hinson, J. M., & Nusbaum, A. T. (2019, April 10). *A dynamic attentional control framework for understanding sleep deprivation effects on cognition.* Progress in brain research. Retrieved January 11, 2023, from https://pubmed.ncbi.nlm.nih.gov/31072558/

37 Saletin, J. M., Goldstein-Piekarski, A. N., Greer, S. M., Stark, S., Stark, C. E., & Walker, M. P. (2016, February 24). *Human hippocampal structure: A novel biomarker predicting mnemonic vulnerability to, and recovery from, sleep deprivation.* Journal of Neuroscience. Retrieved January 11, 2023, from https://www.jneurosci.org/content/36/8/2355#sec-15

38 Pacheco, D., & Wright, H. (2022, September 29). *The best temperature for sleep: Advice & tips.* Sleep Foundation. Retrieved January 11, 2023, from https://www.sleepfoundation.org/bedroom-environment/best-temperature-for-sleep

Chapter 8

39 Moria, T. (2021, June 14). *Throwback: "The crawl" was one of most bizarre triathlon finishes ever.* Triathlon Today. Retrieved January 11, 2023, from https://tri-today.com/2021/06/throwback-the-crawl-as-one-of-most-bizarre-triathlon-finishes-ever/

40 Mavis, B. (2020, December 31). *Recalled: A dramatic duel at the 1997 Hawaii Ironman.* Triathlete. Retrieved January 11, 2023, from https://www.triathlete.com/events/ironman/recalled-a-dramatic-duel/

41 Meeusen, R. (2013, May). *Exercise, nutrition and the brain.* Gatorade Sports Science Institute. Retrieved January 13, 2023, from https://www.gssiweb.org/sports-science-exchange/article/sse-112-exercise-nutrition-and-the-brain

42 MacCormack, J. K., & Lindquist, K. A. (2019, March 19). *Feeling hangry? When hunger is conceptualized as emotion.* Emotion (Washington, D.C.). Retrieved January 11, 2023, from https://pubmed.ncbi.nlm.nih.gov/29888934/

43 Sifferlin, A. (2018, June 11). *Here's why you get hangry, according to science.* Time. Retrieved January 11, 2023, from https://time.com/5307993/heres-why-you-get-hangry/

44 Digestive Health Team, & Lee, C. (2021, December 27). *Is being 'hangry' really a thing or just an excuse?* Cleveland Clinic. Retrieved January 11, 2023, from https://health.clevelandclinic.org/is-being-hangry-really-a-thing-or-just-an-excuse/

45 Bushman, Brad J., Dewall, C. N., Pond Jr., R. S., & Hanus, M. D. (2014, April 29). *Low glucose relates to greater aggression in married couples.* Proceedings of the National Academy of Sciences of the United States of America. Retrieved January 11, 2023, from https://pubmed.ncbi.nlm.nih.gov/24733932/

46 Wittbrodt, M. T., & Millard-Stafford, M. (2018, November). *Dehydration impairs cognitive performance: A meta-analysis : Medicine & science in sports & exercise.* Medicine & Science in Sports & Exercise. Retrieved January 11, 2023, from https://journals.lww.com/acsm-msse/Fulltext/2018/11000/Dehydration_Impairs_Cognitive_Performance__A.21.aspx

47 Bhandari, S. (2021). *Food for concentration: 11 foods that boost memory & help you focus*. WebMD. Retrieved January 11, 2023, from https://www.webmd.com/add-adhd/ss/slideshow-brain-foods-that-help-you-concentrate

48 Jennings, K.-A., & Warwick, K. W. (2021, June 21). *11 best foods to boost your brain and memory*. Healthline. Retrieved January 11, 2023, from https://www.healthline.com/nutrition/11-brain-foods

49 Mathis, A., & Ball, J. (2021, October 5). *6 foods you should be eating every day for better brain health, according to a dietitian*. EatingWell. Retrieved January 11, 2023, from https://www.eatingwell.com/article/7920294/foods-to-eat-every-day-for-brain-health/

50 Hipp, D., & Heyn, P. C. (2023, January 6). *The Best Food for Brain Health*. Forbes. Retrieved January 11, 2023, from https://www.forbes.com/health/healthy-aging/best-brain-food/

51 Axe, J. (2022, July 15). *15 brain foods to boost focus and memory*. Dr. Axe. Retrieved January 11, 2023, from https://draxe.com/nutrition/15-brain-foods-to-boost-focus-and-memory/

52 Naidoo, U. (2022, March 13). *A Harvard nutritionist shares the 6 best brain foods: 'Most people aren't eating enough of' these*. CNBC. Retrieved January 11, 2023, from https://www.cnbc.com/2022/03/12/harvard-nutritionist-shares-the-best-brain-boosting-foods-you-are-not-eating-enough-of.html

53 Kashouty, R. (2021, June 29). *These 10 foods can boost your brain function and neurological health*. Premier Neurology & Wellness Center. Retrieved January 11, 2023, from https://premierneurologycenter.com/blog/10-foods-that-improve-brain-health/

Chapter 9

54 Suttie, J. (2016, March 2). *How nature can make you kinder, happier, and more creative*. Greater Good Magazine. Retrieved January 11, 2023, from https://greatergood.berkeley.edu/article/item/how_nature_makes_you_kinder_happier_more_creative

55 Norwood, M. F., Lakhani, A., Maujean, A., Zeeman, H., Creux, O., & Kendall, E. (2019, July 6). *Brain activity, underlying mood and the environment: A systematic review*. Journal of Environmental Psychology. Retrieved January 11, 2023, from https://www.sciencedirect.com/science/article/abs/pii/S0272494419302397

56 Bratman, G. N., Hamilton, J. P., Hahn, K. S., Daly, G. C., & Gross, J. J. (2015, June 29). *Nature experience reduces rumination and subgenual prefrontal cortex activation*. *PNAS*. Research Article - Psychological and cognitive sciences. Retrieved January 11, 2023, from https://www.pnas.org/doi/10.1073/pnas.1510459112

57 Jimenez, M.P., DeVille N.V., Elliott E.G., Schiff J.E., Wilt G.E., Hart J.E., James P. (2021, April 30) Associations between Nature Exposure and Health: A Review of the Evidence. *International Journal of Environmental Research and Public Health*; 18(9):4790. Retrieved January 11, 2023, from https://doi.org/10.3390/ijerph18094790

58 White, M. P., Alcock, I., Grellier, J., Wheeler, B. W., Hartig, T., Warber, S. L., Bone, A., Depledge, M. H., & Fleming, L. E. (2019, June 13). *Spending at least 120 minutes a week in nature is associated with good health and wellbeing*. Nature News. Retrieved January 11, 2023, from https://www.nature.com/articles/s41598-019-44097-3

Chapter 10

59 Lovering, C., & Diaz, V. (2021, January 13). *Your FAQs answered: Computer eye strain*. Healthline. Retrieved January 11, 2023, from https://www.healthline.com/health/dry-eye/computer-eye-strain

60 Vioguard. (2021, June 1). *93% of young people admit to using their phones on the toilet according to new survey*. 93% of Young People Admit to Using Their Phones on the Toilet According to New Survey. Retrieved January 11, 2023, from https://www.prnewswire.com/news-releases/93-of-young-people-admit-to-using-their-phones-on-the-toilet-according-to-new-survey-301302005.html

61 Ali, T. (2019, June 12). *40% of Aussies use their smartphone in the bathroom*. New Idea. Retrieved January 10, 2023, from https://www.newidea.com.au/smartphone-overuse-in-oz

62 Garten, A. (2019, September 10). *What is the difference between meditation and mindfulness?* Muse. Retrieved January 11, 2023, from https://choosemuse.com/blog/difference-between-meditation-mindfulness/

63 Keim, K. (n.d.). *4 reasons every athlete should meditate*. Headspace. Retrieved January 11, 2023, from https://www.headspace.com/articles/4-reasons-every-athlete-should-meditate

64 Clark, G. (2021, May 21). *The Great Big Multitasking Myth: Why it makes you less efficient*. Deakin University. Retrieved January 11, 2023, from https://this.deakin.edu.au/self-improvement/the-great-big-multitasking-myth-why-it-makes-you-less-efficient

Conclusion

65 Dennehy, C. (2021, November 2). *The simple life of the world's best marathoner*. Runner's World. Retrieved January 15, 2023, from https://www.runnersworld.com/news/a20793538/the-simple-life-of-one-of-the-worlds-best-marathoners/

66 Mackie, J. (2019, October 10). *Can the world's greatest marathoner break the*

two-hour barrier? Runner›s World. Retrieved January 15, 2023, from https://www.
runnersworld.com/uk/training/marathon/a29364019/kipchoge-inoes-159-challenge/

67 Dennehy, C. (2019, September 23). *Not done yet: Kipchoge is ready to defend
his London title.* Runner's World. Retrieved January 15, 2023, from https://www.
runnersworld.com/uk/news/a27235601/kipchoge-is-ready-to-defend-his-london-title/

68 Challenge, I. N. E. O. S. 1:59. (2019, July 4). *"My average sleeping hours is 10 hours.
I sleep for eight hours at night, and two during the day" .You asked him and @
EliudKipchoge answered. Did your #AskEliud questions make the cut? pic.twitter.com/
r7ogkfuugu.* Twitter. Retrieved January 15, 2023, from https://twitter.com/ineos159/
status/1146796221958369280

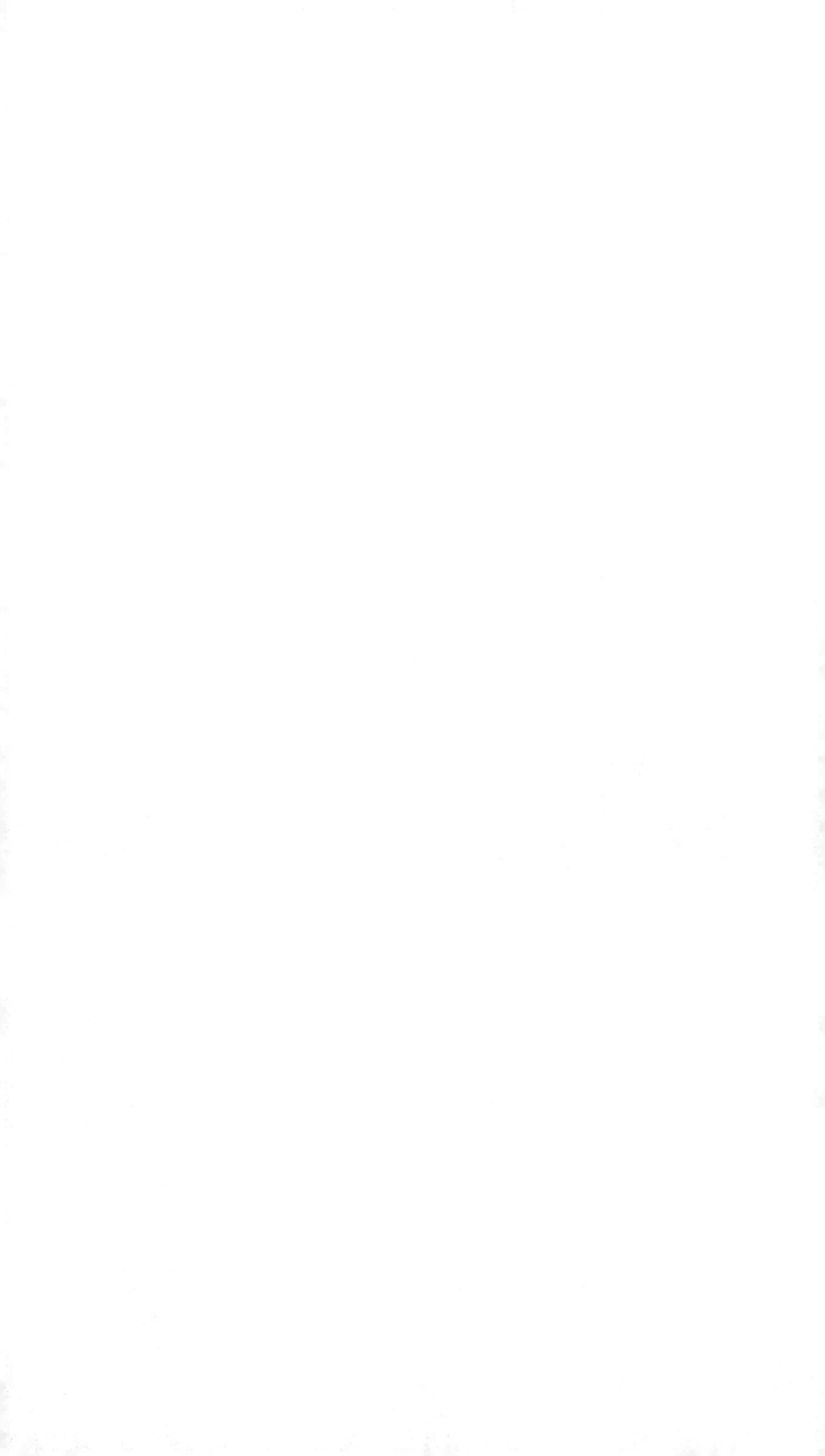